Growing Up with
Bach Flower Remedies

Also by Judy Howard

The Bach Flower Remedies Step by Step

Bach Flower Remedies For Women

Growing Up with Bach Flower Remedies

A GUIDE TO THE USE OF THE REMEDIES DURING CHILDHOOD AND ADOLESCENCE

by Judy Howard

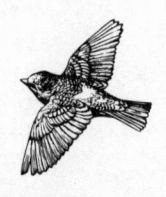

SAFFRON WALDEN
THE C.W. DANIEL COMPANY LIMITED

First published in Great Britain in 1994
by The C.W. Daniel Company Limited
1 Church Path, Saffron Walden
Essex, CB10 1JP, England

© Judy Howard 1994

ISBN 0 85207 273 2

This book is printed on part-recycled paper

Designed by Tim McPhee
Produced in association with
Book Production Consultants Plc, Cambridge
Typeset in New Baskerville
by Cambridge Photosetting Services
and printed by St Edmundsbury Press,
Bury St Edmunds, Suffolk

TO
Alexandra Ellen Ball
and
Katharine Penford Rankin

With a big 'thank you' to
the children of Ollerton
and
Mair Gande, my Fieldwork Teacher and friend
who taught me so much

Contents

Introduction

BACH FLOWER REMEDIES is a well respected system of healing that has been used world-wide since it was established in 1936. The Remedies are natural, entirely safe and children everywhere have benefited enormously from their effects.

The Remedies were discovered by Dr. Edward Bach, a Harley Street physician of very high regard. Having qualified in 1912, he dedicated his life to searching for a system of healing that would be safe, free from side-effects and simple to use. His research took him into bacteriology, immunology and homoeopathy, but having made a thorough study of human nature during the course of his career, he became increasingly convinced that a new system of healing lay within Nature, a system of healing that would bring about natural equilibrium, and heal the conflict between body, mind and spirit which he strongly believed to be the true cause of physical and mental disharmony, thereby relieving suffering by treating the person rather than the disease, and the cause rather than the effect.

Dr. Bach left his medical work in 1930 and went in search of the healing plants of the countryside. One by one, he discovered 38 harmless remedies, each prepared from a different plant, except for one which is prepared from the water of a natural healing spring. The discovery took him over six years to complete, during which time he suffered a variety of mental states and sometimes physical symptoms to help him in his understanding of the healing properties of each plant. It was, at times, an arduous journey, but one he felt privileged to travel, because it enabled him to give to mankind what he earnestly wanted to provide – peace of mind, happiness and health.

Each remedy is for a different emotion, mood or personality and because they cover all states of mind, either individually or in combination, the remedies comprise a timeless system that will help everyone, no matter where they live or into which era they have been born. Society and the pace of life changes with time, but human nature remains the same, and it is this – the emotional outlook – for which the remedies are intended.

In 1934, Dr. Bach made his home in the Oxfordshire village of Sotwell, and lived in a small cottage called Mount Vernon where his work has been continued since his death. Just as he knew precisely when his work began and what he had to do, he knew exactly when it was finished, and when the time came, declared his work to be complete, and asked his trusted colleagues and friends, Nora Weeks and Victor Bullen, to ensure that it remained intact as a system of healing in its own right. His wishes have been upheld by the Dr. Bach Centre at Mount Vernon ever since, ensuring that the Bach Flower Remedies are prepared correctly and carefully, and that the work as a whole retains its hall-mark of purity and simplicity.

My background is in nursing. I commenced my general nurse training in 1977, and later trained and qualified as a midwife. That was a wonderful time of my life as it gave me the opportunity to bring several new babies into the world and is a period that will always have a special place in my memory. I then trained and qualified as a Health Visitor in Nottingham and gained valuable experience with babies and young children of all backgrounds and abilities whilst working in the mining village of Ollerton. Having joined the Dr. Edward Bach Centre at Mount Vernon in 1985, I am privileged to have been taught and guided by my father John Ramsell who worked alongside Dr. Bach's partners, Nora Weeks and Victor Bullen for many years, having been chosen as their successor, and who had a wealth of first hand experience to pass on.

My nursing background and experience as a midwife and Health Visitor, as well as my close involvement with the Bach Flower Remedies has, I hope, enabled me to produce a book that will be of benefit to those with children of their own and anyone else who either works with, looks after or has an active interest in the care of the young.

Each chapter is devoted to a particular period in a child's life, beginning with infancy and ending with young adulthood. Where possible I have referred to "children" rather than "girls and boys", but there are a number of occasions when I have had to resort to the singular and so in many instances have mentioned "him", simply because it would be monotonous and intrusive to the general flow of the book to have to read "him or her" repeatedly. Any reference to "him" or "his", therefore, refers to both girls and boys!

Growth and development is considered, together with the various milestones and stages which potentially – and usually invariably – cause an upheaval of one sort or another. The emphasis, therefore will be on the difficulties associated with growing up because this is when the remedies would be needed the most, but of course there will be just as many good and happy moments, and with the help of the remedies there will be even more!

"*A small child has decided to paint the picture of a house in time for a mother's birthday. In her little mind the house is already painted; she knows what it is to be like down to the very smallest detail, there remains only to put it on paper. To the best of her ability she has put her idea of a house into form. It is a work of art because it is all her very own, every stroke done out of love for her mother, every window, every door painted in with the conviction that it is meant to be there. Even if it looks like a haystack, it is the most perfect house that has ever been painted: it is a success because the little artist has put her whole heart and soul, her whole being into doing of it. This is health, this is success and happiness and true service. Serving through love in perfect freedom in our own way.*

If however, someone came along and said 'why not put a window here, and a door there; and of course the garden path should go this way', the result in the child will be complete loss of interest in the work; she may become cross, irritated, unhappy, afraid to refuse these suggestions; begin to hate the picture and perhaps tear it up: in fact, according to the type of child, so will be the reaction. The final picture may be a recognisable house, but it is an imperfect one and a failure because it is the interpretation of another's thoughts, not the child's. This is disease, the reaction to interference. This is temporary failure and unhappiness: and this occurs when we allow others to interfere with our purpose in life and implant in our minds doubt, or fear, or indifference."

Edward Bach

CHAPTER 1

The Bach System and How It Relates to Children

DR. BACH'S PHILOSOPHY is based on the principle that if we can be ourselves and do what makes us happy, then we will not only reap the benefits of a fulfilling and rewarding life, but also be governors of our own destiny. The quote opposite explains how a child's innocence, if left undisturbed, will blossom and generate all the positive aspects of life, but how, in contrast, that uninhibited freedom and true sense of purpose can so easily be sapped or stifled if negativity is allowed to take control. Happiness, therefore, means living our own life, true to our own convictions. Doing what other people tell us to do, or living and working in accordance with someone else's desires, means we live *their* life, not our own, and just like the child who lost interest in her painting, life itself may become dull and uninteresting, and as a result, our health and happiness can so easily suffer.

The Bach Remedies offer a gentle means of relieving negative attitudes, and because they are prepared from flowers and trees, none of which are poisonous, they provide a harmless, non-habit forming system of healing. One may wonder how something so simple can offer such remarkable benefits, but everything in nature has its own special part to play in the great workings of life. There are a great many homoeopathic, herbal and orthodox medicines derived from plants, and the Bach Remedy flowers hold certain, very special, healing properties too. Some medicines combat physical disorders; the Bach Remedies treat the personality and emotional upset such as impatience, fear and sadness. Dr. Bach believed that negative states such as these, were ultimately responsible for disease, and so treatment of the *underlying* cause, was vital. The Remedies therefore are chosen in accordance with the person's mood and general nature, an approach that gently re-establishes inner equilibrium which gives the body freedom to begin its own natural healing.

I | THE INDICATIONS FOR THE 38 REMEDIES & RESCUE REMEDY

Some remedies describe personalities or character traits. These are the *"type remedies"*. Others are descriptive of more general moods and emotions. These are the *"mood remedies"*. Some are a mixture of the two. When considering which remedy to choose, always consider the child's natural disposition and choose a remedy that best suits his or her personality – i.e. a *"type"* remedy. It is the *"type remedy"* that is the key to the inner balance because it is the child's individuality that determines the response to potentially stressful situations. In addition, however, remedies for the moods can be added, or taken separately, depending on the particular problems the child is facing or a change in the temperament that is the result of external pressure or of feeling unwell.

You will notice that some of the remedy traits describe positive qualities and attitudes. Remedies are not required all the time and it is not necessary to give a happy, contented child a remedy simply because his or her personality fits a description. The remedies will not alter the child's basic constitution, but instead, bring about a return of equilibrium when a child is upset, unsettled or unwell.

❊ A. TYPE REMEDIES

The remedies in this section are those associated with personality traits. They may, however, be required by *any* child should he or she be in the frame of mind described.

AGRIMONY
The Agrimony child has a sunny and outwardly cheerful disposition – a happy child who laughs and always seems to be in good humour. Because the child hides his feelings behind a facade, it is not obvious that he is distressed. The Agrimony remedy will help such children to release their inner turmoil, share it and let it go. It

therefore soothes, brings comfort and a return of the child's natural happiness.

BEECH
Beech children find it hard to be tolerant towards other children. They have an inner belief that *their* way is the *right* way, whether at play, hobbies or at school. Beech children may complain to their parents that another child is not doing something correctly, or may get annoyed with playmates who cannot grasp a certain method. They are not necessarily bad-tempered but may frown on those they consider stupid. As they get older, they may express their intolerance through sarcasm and rebellion. The remedy will help them develop a more sympathetic understanding of others.

CENTAURY
The Centaury child has a placid and generous nature. He finds it hard to stand up for himself and may become the victim of school bullies. At play, Centaury children are happy to share and will show a great deal of care for their toys, playing quietly and non-aggressively. They are "good" children, always doing as they are told.

CERATO
Cerato children are frequently asking "am I doing this right?" because they doubt their judgement. In the classroom they may seek the advice of classmates, copy what they do, or even "cheat" in exams – not because they do not know the answer, but because they want to make sure that their answer is correct. Cerato children can be easily influenced and sometimes misguided because they tend to mimic those they look up to, begin to dress, speak and act like them, and thus risk losing sight of their own personality and identity. The remedy helps these children to know their own mind, to trust in their own beliefs and follow their intuition.

CHICORY
Chicory children are loving and caring and seek similar affection from parents, relatives and friends. They like to see their efforts appreciated and do not like to be ignored. Because of this they have a tendency to "cling", or try to attract attention by making a fuss if

3

there is a threat to their mother's (usually) undivided attention. They may display their negative side by selfishly keeping toys to themselves, unwilling to share playthings. At worst they can be manipulative and possessive, but the positive side of their character is that of a guardian, instinctively looking after a younger child like a mother would look after her baby.

CLEMATIS

Clematis children are daydreamers; those who get "lost" in creativity; those with vivid imaginations who become absorbed in play-acting and imaginary games with imaginary friends. It is this artistic side of the Clematis nature that is the positive expression, but at times, this creativity may become blocked due to lack of concentration, future fantasies and a mind that sometimes wanders aimlessly and blankly. The Clematis remedy helps these children channel their imagination so that instead of being diffused into oblivion, it is a free-flowing, fulfilling expression of the deeply inquisitive and thoughtful Clematis mind.

CRAB APPLE

These children are fussy about detail, and exceptionally neat and tidy, getting upset if toys or clothes are out of order or dirty, and showing a dislike for playing in dirty places. If wet and muddy they will want to be changed into clean clothes immediately. The older Crab Apple child will take care to keep his or her bedroom tidy, fold clothes neatly and so on. Crab Apple children and adults dislike illness intensely and hate being sick, or suffering with upset bowels. The Crab Apple remedy, however, being the cleanser, is important in illness for us all, and not only for those with a Crab Apple nature.

ELM

Elm is the remedy for those who are usually confident but become overwhelmed by an unusual amount of pressure or responsibility. In childhood, this may be when the child, or teenager, is moved into a higher grade. Having scored top marks at one level and so raised to a higher class, he flounders because he feels unable to cope with the more complicated study material and work that is expected of him. Examination times may also create this momentary lack of confidence and when under pressure, can cause panic at the thought of being unable to cope. The Elm remedy helps to revive faith in the child's ability to handle pressure.

HEATHER
Heather children, if they are ill or have suffered an injury, become obsessed with their body and what is wrong with it, describing every ache and pain in detail. Heather children, like Heather adults, are chatterboxes, but this in itself does not necessarily mean that Heather is the appropriate remedy. Many other remedy types have a lot to say as well. If however, the talkativeness is a factor of self-interest, then Heather would be indicated.

IMPATIENS
The traits of Impatiens children are demonstrated in play and social behaviour. They are easily bored and get annoyed if unable to do something quickly enough. They become agitated if another child is hindering them and "itch" to get hold of a thing and do it them-selves. They are excitable and restless children and run around at top speed if something happens to interrupt normal routine (such as visitors coming, having a party, or preparing to go on holiday). At school they are quick minded and are often the first to put up their hand in class, bouncing up and down in their seat eager to demonstrate or provide the answer.

Impatiens babies are restless, irritable, sleep lightly for short periods and may toss and turn in the night.

The remedy is often combined with Vervain as both remedies are indicative of active, highly strung, alert children.

LARCH
Larch children lack self-confidence, and are those who sit quietly in class, for even though they may know the answer, prefer to leave it to someone else to avoid the risk of making a fool of themselves. Larch children fear failure and so would feel far too self-conscious to speak out or take part in a demonstration or sporting activity that has expectations of success. For this reason, Mimulus often complements Larch because as Mimulus is the remedy to ease fear,

shyness and nervousness, it assists the Larch child's search for courage to take that step forward.

MIMULUS
Mimulus is the remedy for fear of people and other known things, so Mimulus children are shy and timid. They tend to blush easily and may be frightened of teachers and older children. The positive side of the Mimulus nature is one of quiet courage, and because they know what it is like to be afraid, to blush and be stuck for words, they develop a depth of understanding for others who are facing similar difficulties.

OAK
Oak children will be the ones who are easily able to shrug things off. If they should become ill they will tend to disregard their ill-health as much as possible and not make a fuss. They are those to whom other children turn, and may become the "agony aunt" (or uncle) of the classroom! They will lead when required, but do not have the bossy or domineering manner of the Vine personality. The Oak prefers to guide, assist and support. The Oak personality is very positive, but has a tendency to overwork and may then become exhausted. It is when the inner strength begins to wane that the remedy is needed.

PINE
Pine children have an apologetic personality, frequently saying "sorry" and worried they have caused some unfortunate event. Pine children immediately blame themselves and feel desperately guilty despite reassurance that they are not to blame. The remedy helps to release the guilty conscience so that they realise that what goes wrong is not necessarily their fault.

RED CHESTNUT
Red Chestnut is a remedy for those who are over anxious about the welfare of others. The Red Chestnut child worries about the welfare of parents, afraid they will have an accident or that a minor illness will develop into a life-threatening disease. The safety, well-being and happiness of animals, friends and other members of the family

are also a source of anxiety, and the Red Chestnut remedy helps put these fears into perspective.

ROCK WATER
Rock Water is the remedy for those who set high standards and are highly self-disciplined. Rock Water children demand perfection in their work and may appear tense in their determination to get everything right. Rock Water children may reprimand themselves if their homework is wrong, and always strive to do better. This is no bad thing, but if it causes mental rigidity, tension, lack of sleep, stress and strain, Rock Water is the remedy to help ease the pressure, and help the child maintain his high standards, but not at the expense of his health and happiness.

SCLERANTHUS
Scleranthus is helpful for any form of imbalance – dilemmas or indecision as well as travel sickness, vertigo and mood swings. The Scleranthus personality is indecisive, hesitant and uncertain. These children find it difficult to make up their minds about what they want to do or where they want to go, and are forever tossing two ideas around in their mind, or missing out on opportunities due to their inability to decide. The remedy helps to steady these fluctuating thoughts and establish more balance and certainty in the mind.

VERVAIN
In the young child, Vervain traits are often demonstrated in over-activity. They, like Impatiens children, tend to get over-excited, but the Vervain excitement is due to eagerness and enthusiasm rather than impatience. These children may complain about the unfair behaviour of another child but they are unlikely to tell-tales because among the Vervain virtues are honesty and loyalty. They dislike cruelty and will support the victim, whether it be a bullied child or a defenceless animal, and may become angry on such occasions. The Vervain remedy does not remove this protective instinct or take their enthusiastic energy away, but when it causes tension, frustration or restlessness, the remedy re-establishes equilibrium.

VINE
Vine children are strong willed and determined to get their own way! They make good leaders but can be aggressive and order other children around. They "take charge" at school and in their determination to get what they want, may throw a tantrum, stubbornly refusing to "behave". The remedy helps to replace this negatively charged energy with the positive qualities of the Vine nature.

WALNUT
Childhood represents a series of changes during a short period of rapid growth and development. This remedy helps children to adjust to these periods of change and is useful during the prominent milestones – teething, going to school, puberty etc.

The Walnut *personality* knows what he or she wants to do, knows the correct answer to a question or the way to play a certain game, but whose conviction falters and is swayed when an alternative idea or approach is presented to them. They may then be persuaded to do something they do not really want to do. The remedy provides the necessary protection from these influences to enable them to maintain constancy and go their own way.

WATER VIOLET
Water Violet children have a self assured, self-contained quality, making just a few close friends. Children of this nature will play happily by themselves and when unwell, dislike attention and prefer to be left quietly alone. They tend to suffer in silence and may become lonely as a result. It is, however, never very easy to read a Water Violet's thoughts as they give little away, and maintain a certain distance between themselves and others, backing off should anyone try to get too close. Consequently one never *really* gets to know a Water Violet fully. There is always something that remains a mystery.

WILD ROSE
Wild Rose children have an "if you can't beat them, join them" attitude and take things very much as they come, accepting what is in store for them without objection. As they grow up, Wild Rose children do not tend to show very much ambition and are not

interested in pursuing a demanding career. Instead, they prefer to wait and see what happens, with an attitude of indifference. Their positive quality is a calm and contented approach to life.

❧ B. MOOD REMEDIES

The following list of remedies are those that are descriptive of emotions that may apply to *any* type of individual. By relieving these negative states of mind, they assist the action of the type remedy in re-establishing equilibrium, and are also useful as remedies in their own right for passing moods.

All the remedies, even the type remedies, may be required at any time by any type of person, and so all 38 remedies may be considered as "mood remedies". However, listed below are those that deal solely with a state of mind rather than constitution.

ASPEN

As with many adults, children experience the sensation of "butter-flies" in the tummy when, for example, they are about to visit the dentist or sit an examination. Although the cause of the anxiety may be known – fear of pain or failure for example – and would there-fore suggest Mimulus or Larch, there is usually an unknown element to the fear as well – fear of what the dentist *might* do, what the examination paper *might* involve. Aspen is for the sense of appre-hension associated with a vague fear of the unknown and sense of uneasiness for no apparent reason.

CHERRY PLUM

This remedy would help children who are hysterical, delirious or have a sudden impulse to do something out of character. It would also be indicated on occasions when a child may suddenly have an outburst of temper and cease to have any apparent self-control. The action of the remedy is to calm the frightened and diverted thoughts, and bring about a more rational state of mind.

CHESTNUT BUD

Chestnut Bud is the remedy for those who do not learn from ex-perience and so make the same mistake over and over again. Child-hood is a constant learning period and on the whole, children *do* learn. Sometimes they need to experience things more than once before the message really sinks in, but that is probably true for most of us. If, however, a child goes on repeating the same mistakes, Chestnut Bud will help him appreciate the significance of his experience.

GENTIAN

Gentian is the remedy for those who feel discouraged following a set-back. Children may feel disappointed if they are told they cannot go out to play, or that they are not going to visit "Aunty Pauline" after all, or downhearted because they do not feel well, or depressed because they have lost their favourite toy or broken mum's best vase! When examination time comes, lower marks than expected may cause intense disappointment, as would being told they are not suitable for the school sports team. Gentian would be indicated on all these occasions and helps children to face similar situations, if and when they occur in the future, more positively.

GORSE

The true Gorse state is not often seen in children because, on the whole, they have such a fresh appetite for life that the hopeless pessimism of Gorse is not often apparent. However, there may be occasions when the remedy is required, perhaps during a major crisis at home or after failed examinations, when they lose the inclination to try again. If a child or young person should lose hope, Gorse is the remedy to help the sparkle re-appear.

HOLLY

Holly is for envy, hatred, suspicion and the desire for revenge. In children it would include spitefulness, bullying, pinching, biting etc., as well as jealousy of other children's friends, toys or family. Holly will help the child, whatever the object of his feelings, to be less "angry" and more able to get along peaceably with other children.

HONEYSUCKLE

This remedy is for those who dwell on the past. Children are generally keen, and focused on what is going on *now*, and so are not likely to become absorbed with thoughts of the past to this extent.

There are however, occasions when the remedy is required, for example, if a child suffers a trauma and the memory plays on his or her mind, haunting the sleep. Or if a child has lost a parent or grandparent and the grief causes constant reflection, sometimes trying so hard to remember every detail, that interest in the present slips away. Honeysuckle is also indicated for homesickness and would therefore help children when they go on a school trip and are parted from their parents or home for a while.

HORNBEAM
This remedy is for procrastination and the kind of weariness that occurs *before* something happens. It is generally the thought of what is about to happen or of what one has to do, that causes this feeling of lethargy; something that may be encountered before school, especially if there is a lesson that day which the child does not like. Children may also feel this way at the thought of doing their homework, washing their hair or having a bath, suddenly overcome with a sense of fatigue and wish to "do it later". The energy however, miraculously seems to return if a friend should call round and something more interesting is on offer! The remedy helps to provide the strength to face what lies ahead, so that routine and seemingly mundane duties become more of a pleasure than a chore, and activities – even homework! – become interesting rather than monotonous.

MUSTARD
This remedy is for the sort of depression that descends for no particular reason. Usually there is a reason for a child's depression, in which case Gentian might be more appropriate, but sometimes it descends like a dark cloud, as if from nowhere, and is more common during puberty and adolescence than in young children.

OLIVE
This remedy is for tiredness – *genuine* tiredness due to overwork. It may be required at examination time for mental fatigue after an excess amount of study. Tiredness is also likely to occur due to frequent late nights, although the best remedy for *this* is sleep! The remedy can be helpful if the child is recovering from illness, when

the body has naturally become depleted of energy, and can assist during the convalescent period to hasten a return to health.

ROCK ROSE

This remedy is for terror, great fear, something that may cause panic. In childhood the remedy can be particularly helpful for nightmares. There are, however, many occasions when children may become terrified – they may have seen or imagined something or heard a horror story that has frightened them so much that it has created panic and terror. Any occasion when the fear is much greater than nervousness (for which Mimulus would be more appropriate), Rock Rose would be helpful.

STAR OF BETHLEHEM

This remedy would be helpful for children who have suffered a shock or bereavement, and feel sad and lonely as a result. Star of Bethlehem would help them to cope with the sadness of their loss. The shock of a fall, accident or of being startled by something are also occasions when Star of Bethlehem would be helpful (but see also Rescue Remedy).

SWEET CHESTNUT

This remedy is for a deep sense of anguish; despair as though life is no longer worthwhile. It is not often that you will see children in the true depths of the Sweet Chestnut state, but it would be a helpful remedy for the occasions when they should feel heartbroken, for example should they lose a pet which has become as loyal and true as any friend, or person whom they love. It would, on occasions such as this, work hand-in-hand with Star of Bethlehem to relieve the grief. It is also helpful during the teenage years when despair is more often experienced. The remedy soothes and comforts and helps the despair to lift so that something brighter appears on the horizon and shows them that all is not lost.

WHITE CHESTNUT

This remedy is indicated for persistent worrying thoughts which may cause restlessness and sleepless nights. Worry over schoolwork, forth-coming examinations, visiting the dentist, presenting some work in class, the expected back-lash having misbehaved... are all occasions when White Chestnut would be helpful.

WILD OAT
This remedy is for those who have ambition and desire to do something worthwhile, but feel lost as to which direction to take. The most likely time young people would need Wild Oat would be when they are required to make a decision about their future and the career they should follow. The remedy helps by clearing the confusion so they can see which way they want to go.

WILLOW
This remedy is for resentment, bitterness and self-pity, and for those who feel life has treated them unfairly. Willow helps those who find it hard to forgive and forget. Children may feel resentful towards parents who have reason not to allow them to go out to play, or towards school-friends for playing a trick or breaking a friendship. The remedy would also help children who sulk when told off, seek sympathy or try to make others feel guilty by bursting into tears. It is for the "huff" and other introspective moods. The action of the remedy is to bring the lighter side of life back into focus, to promote optimism and allow the thoughts to be cast outward rather than inward, thus accepting blame where it is due, being able to say sorry and forgive more readily.

RESCUE REMEDY
This is a combination of five of the 38 remedies. It is intended for emergencies – accidents, alarm, examination nerves and so on, occasions when there is a degree of shock or panic causing a person to feel suddenly shaken and disturbed. It consists of the following:

STAR OF BETHLEHEM – for shock
ROCK ROSE – for terror
CHERRY PLUM – for panic and hysteria
CLEMATIS – for feeling faint or stunned
IMPATIENS – for the agitation and irritation that is so often associated with pain.

Rescue Remedy as a liquid is ideal for situations as described above and would be taken orally to calm the troubled mind. Rescue Remedy Cream is helpful for external trauma such as bumps, bruises, cuts and grazes. It is soothing and helps to promote healing, and also contains CRAB APPLE for its cleansing properties.

Rescue Remedy and its uses specifically in relation to children will be discussed in more detail a little further on in this chapter.

II | **SELECTING REMEDIES FOR CHILDREN**

The treatment of adults is often considered to be much easier than that of children because adults are, usually, able to express their emotions, describe how they feel, know their personality and the cause of their unhappiness. To help an adult we simply need to sit down and have a two-way conversation – the one needing help opening up and talking freely about his or her feelings, and the other asking the relevant questions to elucidate or clarify the correct remedy or remedies that may be required. It is not possible to have this kind of frank discussion on the same level with very young children, and because of this, the Bach Remedies are sometimes regarded as being of little help to them, which is unfortunate because the remedies can help very much indeed. In fact, children respond to the remedies, on the whole, far quicker than adults, so the inner balance is re-established much sooner and much more easily. Children are fresh, innocent, new to this world of experience, and so do not have a lifetime of accumulated frustrations and upsets interfering with their outlook on life. The remedies when needed, can set about helping them straight away, unhindered, and without having to fight their way through an assault course of barriers and influences first. We are rather like an onion – beginning as a small bulb, but as we get older, and bigger, layer upon layer builds up around us so that eventually the little bulb in the middle may become overwhelmed or even lost beneath all the outer layers and tough skin. The remedies are there to help us peel back those layers so that our true personality can emerge once more, free to express itself, grow and develop in its own right. Because a child is only a small "onion" – still only that little bulb –

the remedies get to work and combat the problem much more quickly.

In choosing remedies for children, we need to not only take notice of what they say, but how they behave, how they mix with other children or interact with adults, how they play – are they able to amuse themselves or do they get bored easily? Do they become frustrated when they cannot draw a picture properly or build the bricks in a straight line, or do they patiently try again? We need to consider their behaviour, their mood and personality in these terms, and compare the negative behaviour with the child's normal or usual behaviour. For example, if a child is usually outgoing and boisterous, but suddenly becomes introverted and timid, then not only should we consider the reasons for this change, which may be related to fear in this instance, we should also take into account the child's natural outgoing personality. Remedies for both these things therefore would be chosen to bring about a complete balance.

Even at a very young age, babies will display unique characteristics – perhaps in the way they cry, the way they move, hold their heads, respond to sight and sound and so on. Even tiny babies can get in a temper if they are hungry or need changing, and if their needs are not interpreted correctly, they will soon let you know! Some babies are quicker off the mark in this respect than others – some are quick tempered, yelling at the top of their voices; others are passive and will only cry if they really have to, merely murmering to attract your attention; some babies will let you put them in their cot without a sound, grinning contentedly at you, happy to gaze around until sleep overcomes them; others do not want to be alone, will only be quiet when picked up, get over-tired and resist sleep. They are all different and so it is their individual character that needs to be considered when choosing the remedies to help them. For the contented baby that never seems to complain, who is never any "trouble", CENTAURY would be appropriate, or WILD ROSE for the more impartial child. The baby who wants to be picked up and constantly cuddled would indicate CHICORY; the baby who has a short temper would benefit from IMPATIENS; the baby who gurgles happily even when he or she has a dirty nappy would be an AGRIMONY baby.

As the months pass, the infant's personality and individuality will develop more and more, just as the child's physical growth takes place. Milestones are reached in physical, social and psychological development, and are common to all children, although each one retains an individuality throughout life which will establish a unique character.

Ups and downs are important learning experiences, vital for the child's emotional development. The Bach Remedies do not deny the child the opportunity to learn, but sometimes awkward and difficult periods, experiences and situations may, instead of *aiding* emotional development, hinder its progress by making the child *too* frightened, *too* withdrawn or *too* unhappy. The remedies are not a crutch or an easy option, but are there to help children reach that delicate balance for themselves, and are therefore like fuel for the mind, just as food is fuel for the body.

III | **ADMINISTERING THE REMEDIES TO CHILDREN**

All the Bach Remedy plants are non-poisonous, and by virtue of the way the remedies are made, entirely harmless. No part of the plant is actually ingested – it is only the healing energy that forms the active ingredient. Something intangible, but nonetheless effective. The only added ingredient is brandy which acts as a preservative. It is the brandy content that often causes a few questions as to the remedies' suitability for children.

Brandy forms the bulk of the "stock" remedy – that is, the concentrated remedy. However, stock remedies are not intended to be taken neat, they should be diluted in water, even for adults. The dilution is as follows:

2 drops of each required stock remedy into a 30ml bottle of water. From this bottle take 4 drops 4 times daily.

The consumption of brandy therefore, taken in each dose, or even each day, is negligible and barely measurable. A number of medicinal preparations contain alcohol because it is a widely used preservative, but because medicines do not normally contain a list of ingredients, it is not always known whether a particular product has an alcohol content or not. It is because the brandy in the Bach Remedies is so *obvious* and not disguised in any way that it raises so many questions. It is, however, as mentioned previously, only the *stock* remedies that contain this quantity of brandy. The stock remedies are taken diluted as described above, and even after this dilution has been made, the dosage drops can be further diluted into a drink if preferred. The remedies benefit children so much that it would be a great shame if their use was rejected simply out of ignorance of the correct method of administration. I hope this explanation will help to reassure those who may be concerned about giving the remedies to children because of the alcohol content. If for any particular reason you *are* worried however, do speak to your Health Visitor or family doctor who will be able to advise you accordingly and put your mind at ease.

Although drops can be administered directly into the child's mouth from the prepared treatment bottle, it is usually more convenient to simply add the drops to a drink of water or fruit juice. The child then does not need to feel that he or she is taking a medicine, although there are many children who enjoy taking their "drops" and take an active interest in them. The remedies can be added to hot drinks too, so if you give a warm drink at bed-time, the evening drops can be taken in that. For babies, prepare the treatment using cooled boiled water, sterilising the bottles as you would the infant's other utensils. If you prefer not to give the remedies to your baby orally, then apply the dilution to the infant's wrists, temples, fontanelles and beneath the ears. Otherwise, simply add the drops to a bottle of milk, water or juice, or offer on a teaspoon. Young babies still being breast-fed will obtain benefit from the remedies if the mother herself takes them as they will find their way into the baby through her milk. Alternatively apply the drops to the nipple so the baby obtains the remedy at the start of a feed, or simply put a few drops into the infant's mouth. One needs to be imaginative in order to find the method that suits you both.

The minimum dosage (from the diluted treatment bottle) is 4 drops 4 times daily which, ideally, should be fairly evenly spaced out – a dose on rising in the morning, a dose when retiring to bed at night and twice during the day, e.g. mid-morning and mid-afternoon. This stipulation often causes parents concern if the child is unable to take the drops whilst at school. Once again, one needs to be flexible, and so a dose may be given in the morning, and then three times during the course of the late afternoon/evening. If this is not possible, then instead of 4 doses of 4 drops (i.e. 16 drops per day), give 2 doses of 8 drops, morning and night. If the child takes a packed lunch to school, then the mid-day drops can be added to a drink or even included in a sandwich! Some children will happily take their drops, whilst others are reluctant. Every child's needs are different, and so once again a little ingenuity is called for to find the best method for *your* child.

| IV | **RESCUE REMEDY IN CHILDHOOD** |

Rescue Remedy is probably the most essential Bach Remedy to have in the house whilst your children are young. It has endless uses and because children seem to attract emergencies of one sort or another, having Rescue Remedy to hand there and then will help enormously. As with all the other Bach Remedies, Rescue Remedy is a liquid and would be taken in water when required. The dosage, however, is 4 drops of the stock remedy in 30ml of water instead of the usual 2. A child who has fallen over and bruised himself or grazed a knee therefore could be given a few drops of Rescue Remedy in a drink to sip, as this would ease the shock and distress, but it can also be applied to the bruise or graze (make sure the liquid stock remedy is diluted as it may otherwise sting), and this will help to relieve the external trauma, and in turn, relieve the pain and distress. The Rescue Remedy Cream is probably even better for cuts and grazes as it contains Crab Apple for its cleansing properties as well as the Rescue Remedy ingredients. It makes a very soothing healing salve and is a "must" for the first aid box – along with the liquid Rescue Remedy of course!

One cannot be too careful where children are concerned, and so although Rescue Remedy is without a doubt, invaluable in an emergency, it does not take the place of medical attention, so if you are at all concerned then do call the doctor. If a more serious accident has occurred – perhaps resulting in the child having hit his head and being knocked unconscious, then whilst awaiting the arrival of the ambulance or doctor, Rescue Remedy can be applied to the wrists, temples, beneath the ears and around the lips, (the remedy will still be effective even though it is not actually ingested), to comfort and aid the healing process. I have heard of several instances following a dose of Rescue Remedy when the child has soon begun playing normally again! Even so, head injuries should *always* be checked medically and I feel sure that any parent would feel more secure in their own mind by the reassurance that no lasting damage had been done.

In young childhood, when the child is still learning to walk, there will be many occasions when the Rescue Remedy will be needed – falls, bumps, bruises etc., are commonplace. Also minor burns and scalds – a hot cup of tea being knocked over for example, would call for some first aid measure. Rescue Remedy diluted with water, dabbed on and left to evaporate will allow the area to cool, and help to relieve the shock and pain so healing can begin straight away. The Cream may also be applied, but only if the burn is superficial and *only* when the initial heat and soreness has subsided as it is not advisable to put cream on a recent burn. Medical attention should always be sought if the burn is severe, and I would advise you to call the doctor if you are in any way concerned – even if it is only for your own peace of mind.

The calming influence that Rescue Remedy has on a young child can be quite outstanding. It is wise therefore to carry it around with you so that it is always readily available, because with young children about, you never know when you are going to need it!

CHAPTER 2

Children's Challenges

CHILDHOOD IS FULL of new challenges and although the passage through the various stages is usually smooth, there are several difficult periods when problems are likely to arise, both for the child and for the parent. In this chapter, we will look at these areas and discuss the difficulties that can take place, with I hope, some helpful suggestions for all concerned.

I | **BIRTH** The first challenge a child faces is being born, and for most babies it is a natural straightforward journey. Occasionally however, birth is a traumatic event with lasting consequences. Prolonged labour, lack of oxygen, and so on, may cause what is termed "foetal distress" and this may mean that certain measures need to be taken to deliver the baby quickly. The procedure taken will depend on local hospital policy or midwifery practice, but may involve an emergency Caesarean section together with resuscitation of the baby if necessary once it has been born. Almost always this emergency treatment quickly gets the situation under control and the baby starts to breathe (or cry!) normally. Nevertheless it is bound to be an immensely traumatic few moments, for the baby as well as the mother and father. STAR OF BETHLEHEM, the remedy for shock, is an important remedy for the relief of such trauma. Star of Bethlehem is one of the ingredients of RESCUE REMEDY which is usually more readily to hand, and is ideal for such occasions. It would help the parents who can sip it from a glass of water, but if possible, a few drops diluted into sterile water could be dabbed around the baby's wrists and temples to help make the transition into this world more comfortable.

The infant has entered a strange new world and has absolutely *everything* to learn and experience. He or she will gradually develop social skills, encounter emotions, discomfort, hunger, thirst, not getting his or her own way... and these learning experiences begin immediately.

BONDING

A baby's eyes cannot focus until about six weeks of age, but he can nevertheless make out shapes, albeit fuzzy shapes, which he gradually learns to relate to and recognise. The mother's hair colour for example will help the baby identify who she is. She will also have a unique smell which the baby will naturally be attracted to, and because bright lights and shiny objects are always those which are most noticeable, standing out from blurry vision, her smile and eye sparkle also attract attention, and the eyes especially become a source of fascination. For the first hours and days, the newborn infant will keep its eyes closed a great deal of the time, but gradually will begin to realise that it is much more interesting to keep them open, and it is then that notice is really taken of his surroundings. Eye to eye contact is extremely important, and during the course of feeding, the baby will look up into his mother's eyes and regard her face intently. The familiar appearance and the sound of her voice become synonymous with the warmth and closeness of feeding at her breast, and the safety of her arms. Bottle fed babies are not deprived of this closeness by any means. They can be held just as closely, with just as much eye contact as those who are breast fed, and so the same reaction and development of warmth will be established. This important "bonding" process between mother and baby develops during the first few days, when the natural chemistry that exists between them is marked by a huge instinctive emotional surge when the baby is born and placed in its mother's arms for the first time. This is not *always* how it is however, and for some mothers, other emotions get in the way of these maternal impulses. Bonding then, may need to be worked at and developed as time goes on, as mother and baby gradually get to know each other.

Throughout Dr. Bach's writings, he emphasises the importance of the emotional outlook and addressing and treating the temperament, personality and moods of the person, regardless of what happened to be the object of distress. It is encouraging to find child psychology experts supporting the same principles in which Dr. Bach so strongly believed. John Bowlby, a child psychiatrist who has researched mother and baby bonding very deeply, believes that emotional development is *the* most important aspect of human (and animal) development.

It is not difficult to appreciate how a closeness develops between mother and baby, but if we separate the link between childbearing and bonding, it is interesting to consider what it is that actually takes place. Looking at it objectively, several questions arise: Is it necessary for a "mother" to be female? Or can fathers be "mothers"? There is really no reason why not, so long as someone fills the role, and one might argue that because bonding begins during pregnancy and culminates in the baby's arrival, it is related to the physical and genetic link between a baby and its natural parents. Adoptive parents, however, also have a fantasy about the baby they will receive so perhaps it is the formation of the image and its revelation that is more crucial to bonding than actually physically bearing the child, because adoptive parents are certainly no less mothering. If anything, they are likely to be *more* doting because the arrival of their baby could be the climax of possibly ten or fifteen years of longing and yearning for a child.

Perhaps, therefore, bonding is a *learned* process and the important thing is consistency, familiarity and recognition through sight, smell and sound. There is, however, one other ingredient – the most vital of all – and that is love. But how can love be measured? It cannot be bottled or inspected under a microscope. It cannot even be properly explained. Sometimes when we think about the remedies and how they work, we may wonder what action and reaction goes on to create their effect. Just like being deeply moved by a certain piece of music, it is difficult to explain, and love is rather like that. We feel it, we recognise it, but cannot explain it, and do not necessarily understand it.

The love bond between mother/father and baby can perhaps be best explained as a sensitivity to one another – a subliminal "tuning in" to each other. Just as we might have a "gut feeling" about something, or have an unexplained awkwardness in a certain person's company, so bonding holds similar messages, and rather like falling in love, we don't question it – we just accept it and enjoy it!

Fathers (the ones who are not "mothers"!) may, understandably, sometimes feel a little left out or disconnected from the cosy routine that mother and child have naturally created. It is, after all, usually the father – husband or partner – who is working during the first weeks and months of his child's life. There are a great number of working mothers but they have the benefit of maternity leave, and are therefore able during this time to establish a close relationship with their baby. It also gives the first time mother time to acquaint herself with "baby-care" techniques so that she feels comfortable when attending to baby's needs. If the father is away at work all day, and asleep all night (if he is lucky!), then he will only be able to spend a few hours with his child, and because he has not had as much time to become well practised, he may feel awkward and clumsy which may lead him to leave it to his wife/partner, making him feel even more isolated. Many dads however do make sure they take an active role in caring for their offspring and take a great deal of interest in all that is concerned with their care, realising the importance of sharing these precious moments. Unfortunately for some fathers, it is not possible, no matter how much they would like it to be, due to work commitments that may take them away from home – those who work aboard ship or long-distance drivers for example – or those who work shifts or longer hours than usual and simply do not have the time. The Bach Remedies cannot bring him home earlier if his job demands a late shift, but they can certainly help him through the many facets of emotions that he may face. OLIVE if he is overworking and getting tired; PINE if he feels guilty for not playing his full part, feels he is neglecting his family or blames himself for his wife's tiredness; HONEYSUCKLE for the man who works for long periods away from home and spends his time counting the days until he is back again; WALNUT for the man who finds the new routine of a baby in the house difficult to adjust to; GENTIAN for the man who feels despondent or depressed with his home or his work; VERVAIN and/or ROCK WATER for men who are workaholics and perfectionists – Vervain for those who are over-enthusiastic, Rock Water for those who force themselves to reach high standards. In both cases, the appropriate remedy helps to relieve the mental and physical tension. For the man who is overwhelmed with the responsibility of having to provide for his new family, ELM would be helpful, and WHITE CHESTNUT for the worried man who tosses and turns at night, thoughts going round and round in his mind...

Mothers may also need help. They too can feel overwhelmed with the responsibility of bringing up a child, responsible for a new life, and so ELM would be indicated for them too. Women also feel despondent (GENTIAN), worried (WHITE CHESTNUT, or RED CHESTNUT if her concern is due to fear over her child's well-being), guilty (PINE), frightened she may lose control (CHERRY PLUM), utterly exhausted (OLIVE), feeling stretched to the limits, desperately unhappy, wishing she could find a way out (SWEET CHESTNUT), or depressed for no reason at all (MUSTARD).

It is, however, as in every case as far as the Bach Remedies are concerned, important to ask *why* you are worried, *why* you are afraid, *why* you are so tired... The answer may be that your baby is not sleeping, or not feeding well, or cries constantly, in which case we should consider remedies to help your baby as well as yourself.

II | **SLEEPING** | Throughout life, sleep is an aspect of living that can, for some people, be a constant source of concern – either having too much sleep, feeling tired or sleepy for much of the day, or not getting enough of it, perhaps suffering with insomnia and unrefreshing sleep. For most people, thankfully, it is a pleasant activity. We all need different amounts of sleep – some people are happy and fully refreshed after only five or six hours, whilst others need at least eight hours to have any hope of functioning normally! Whatever our individual needs might be, it is something that is essential to us all, for without it, insurmountable problems can result.

Sleep is a learned rhythm, and our "in-built clock" is responsible for the correct timing of that rhythm. Anyone who has travelled on a long-haul flight across time zones will be familiar with "jet-lag" and it can take several days before the body reattunes itself to the new rhythm and gets accustomed to a new time pattern.

During a night's sleep, we go through a succession of cycles, each of which lasts about 90 minutes or so. An adult who sleeps for eight hours at night will go through several sleep cycles during that time, and each cycle has five stages. A night's sleep therefore is a period of activity as well as relaxation, and as we will see, there is a lot more to it than one might first assume – a great deal goes on whilst we remain oblivious to it all....

Stage One – Drowsiness
This is the "drifting off" stage, during which time our brain gradually moves from consciousness to unconsciousness, but when we can easily be woken, and sometimes it is a falling sensation or the "floating" feeling when reality becomes confused at the beginning of a dream, that is enough to wake us up.

Stage Two – Greater relaxation
During this period the system is much more relaxed although we may still be woken quite easily by a loud noise or if we are shaken.

Stage Three – Complete relaxation
During this period, the mind and body are totally relaxed. The pulse rate drops and the sleeper cannot be woken by light stimulus alone.

Stage Four– Very deep sleep
The sleeper hardly moves and is very difficult to wake.

Stage Five – The dreaming stage
This is a return to lighter sleep when the brain becomes more active. It is sometimes known as Rapid Eye Movement (R.E.M.) sleep because the eyes move from side to side underneath their lids, rapidly in response to the mental images that form the dream.

A growth hormone is produced during stages 3 and 4, and so when we go through major growth milestones – childhood, adolescence, pregnancy and so on – we will have longer periods of deep sleep. R.E.M. sleep is associated with brain activity, and it is generally more evident during periods of mental stimulation. If there is something playing on our mind, it is likely that we will have prolonged periods of light sleep with associated dreaming, and find it difficult to pass from this superficial brain-active stage into deep sleep, if in fact we get to sleep at all! Hence it becomes unrefreshing and frequently leads to anxiety, resulting in repeatedly disturbed nights.

Children go through the same pattern and stages of sleep as an adult, although as has been said previously, longer periods of deep sleep are natural because so much growth goes on during the early years of life. This is why babies sleep so much. Each baby has its own in-built physiological need for sleep, so some will need, and therefore take, more or less than others. Sometimes we *expect* a baby to sleep all the time, waking only for feeds, and if it does not go to sleep, we fret about the baby's sleeping "problem". However, if a baby does not *need* any more sleep than it is taking, then attempts to settle it down will be in vain! Sometimes therefore, an apparent sleep problem is not a problem for the baby at all. Babies will sleep when they need to, but at the same time, one needs to help them form a rhythm so that they know the difference between night and day. Nevertheless, it is normal for babies to wake during the night for a feed during the first few months. Before they are weaned, this may occur two or three times during the course of the night, but this is natural and normal, and whilst babies are on a milk-only diet, it is important that they *do* wake, especially during the first few weeks. Gradually however, they will settle for longer periods until they sleep right through. Once infants reach about 9 months, they can, to a certain extent, control their sleep and so this is the time when real sleep problems, if there are to be any, usually begin.

❋ COMFORT AND ROUTINE

Getting into a routine from an early age will pay dividends in the long term, making it easier on both yourself and your child as he or she gets older. If the child learns that night is for sleep and daytime is for play, this will help to prevent the night feed becoming a regular playtime. Bed-time rituals – bath, warm drink and a bed-time story or song are relaxing and help to establish an atmosphere conducive to sleep, thereby helping the child learn to distinguish between what is expected of him at night and during the day.

Some children need other forms of comfort – a dummy, "cuddly" blanket or favourite toy for example. They may not feel secure in the dark and so a lamp in the room or a light outside the room will be reassuring and help to allay their fear. Being cuddled is also comforting and very young babies do need this form of contact comfort. Sometimes babies will *only* settle when picked up and nursed. Having explored all other possible reasons for restlessness – hunger, thirst, too hot, cold, uncomfortable etc., you might conclude that the endless crying is for your attention and nothing more. Nevertheless, it can be the hardest thing in the world for a mother to resist the temptation to pick her baby up as soon as it cries. Indeed, knowing what *should* be done is one thing but all logical thought has a habit of suddenly evaporating and being overtaken by panic in a frantic attempt to quieten a tense and agitated baby. Like everything else, it is always easier said than done, and sometimes it is so much easier all round to give in to the child's wishes – anything for a peaceful night!

Occasionally children have more extreme methods of comforting themselves – head banging or rocking. It is important to seek the cause in order to treat the problem and avoid it becoming a habit too difficult to break. There are several reasons, and it is the manifestation in each individual child that determines the appropriate remedy. If the behaviour is a result of fear, then CHERRY PLUM would help restore a more rational control over the impulse to either head-bang or inflict some other form of injury or discomfort; ASPEN for the apprehension that may be felt – the child not really knowing *why* he or she reacts this way, feeling afraid for an unknown reason; MIMULUS for general known fears – fear of being alone, fear of the dark and so on (Aspen might be a helpful addition here as there is often an unknown element to these particular fears). Alternatively, the reason for the behaviour may be *over*-tiredness, in which case OLIVE would be a helpful remedy, but of course it is also important to establish *why* the child is tired and then direct corrective treatment at the cause.

Head-banging, rocking and other forms of comfort behaviour may be the result of something that is worrying the child (WHITE CHESTNUT), or sapping his or her confidence (LARCH). HOLLY would help if the child is jealous – perhaps he feels left out because he believes a sibling is receiving more attention. Another helpful remedy would be CRAB APPLE as this, being the cleansing remedy, would help to free the child from the obsessive self-destructive behaviour. ROCK WATER may also help here to enable the child to relax. STAR OF BETHLEHEM would help to relieve any shock the child might have had, and ROCK ROSE would help to relieve terror should this be apparent. CHICORY would be helpful if the behaviour has become a mechanism for attention, and WALNUT would help the child to adjust and settle. CHESTNUT BUD would help to release him from the repetitiveness, and this, together with Walnut would help him break the habit. The personality of the child, however, should also be considered as this is fundamental to his or her complete treatment – it is, after all, the child's individual character that causes the reaction, so in addition to remedies such as those suggested above for various aspects of the behaviour, the remedy for the child's *type* should be chosen as well.

❦ SLEEP DISTURBANCES

There are endless reasons for children's sleeping difficulties – a problem at school, concern about the imminent arrival of a new brother or sister, or fear of rejection. Children can be very quick to learn how to manipulate, and know that if they cry they will be rewarded with a cuddle, a drink or allowed to join in the evening activities. Disturbed sleep patterns may therefore be an indication of the child's need or desire for attention. Again this may occur because he feels left out, or during a family upheaval such as parents who have separated, or the arrival of a step-parent. When there is something wrong, or when a child is upset or anxious, invariably there is some form of disrupted sleep – frightening dreams, restlessness, uncharacteristic sleepwalking, wakefulness, tearfulness or climbing into bed with parents. The need for attention may cause the child to "cling". CHICORY is the remedy for this. WILLOW would be useful for tearfulness, moaning, whining as though for sympathy, and HEATHER for the child who constantly seeks company. AGRIMONY would help the child who is normally happy and appears to be content during the day yet has restless fretful nights.

Many children are restless because something on their mind

makes them feel uneasy. ASPEN is the remedy to help relieve that apprehension and unknown fear. Some children however, are not upset about anything in particular and are simply lively individuals who wake up early and never seem to be tired in the evening! VERVAIN is the remedy for the type of child who is full of energy, keen to be doing something, perhaps a highly strung child who finds it hard to "wind down" when excited. On these occasions, the child tries to stay awake, resisting sleep, and as a result becomes over-tired which aggravates the whole problem. The Vervain remedy in such a case would help that child to relax so that the system is able to give in to the call for rest and allow sleep to take place with less of a struggle. Other active children may be of the IMPATIENS nature – such children tend to rush about and never sit still, their mind alert and quickly ticking over. This type of child, like the Vervain child, may have difficulty "letting go" of the interest in the moment, fighting the desire to sleep and as the child becomes over-tired, he grows irritable and agitated, short-tempered and impatient. Impatiens therefore helps to relieve this mental tension to enable the child to submit to the beckoning tiredness.

At the other extreme, there are children who seem to be constantly sleepy – yawning during the day, yet sleeping soundly at night. They may be difficult to wake, and have trance-like dreams which may include sleep-walking. CLEMATIS would be the indicated remedy for this and these children may be of the Clematis type; those who tend to day-dream or have difficulty concentrating. Clematis children are usually creative with a vivid imagination into which they will drift, mentally escaping from real life into a world of make-believe. WILD ROSE children are also of this "drowsy" type of temperament, but Wild Roses are more apathetic and go along with the crowd, even though their heart is not always in it. It is the lack of energy and enthusiasm that causes the Wild Rose to seem drowsy, and they will often go to sleep for want of something better to do!

When the infant is ready to move into a cot or into his own room, another set of sleeping problems may arise. Again, there are various theories as to how to make it easier – placing the small cot into the larger one for a while, sleeping in the baby's new bedroom with him until he is happy to sleep alone (could be a long time!), warming the cot so that it seems as cosy as the old one, and so on. You may need to try a number of measures until you find one that suits your own child's needs. As far as the Bach Remedies are concerned, the most appropriate would be WALNUT because it is indicated in times of change and will therefore help the infant to settle into his new environment.

❀ NIGHTMARES

Among the most problematic and common sleep disturbances in childhood are nightmares. These can begin at an early age and may indeed last a lifetime, and occur for a variety of reasons. Fear, however, is a primary cause – fear of the dark or of snakes under the bed, spiders in the bed-clothes, the "bogey-man" and so on. Different situations create different fears. The shapes of the trees against a moon-lit sky, or shapes created by the movement of curtains can play some frightening games with a child's imagination. A child who has woken up to find his mother or father is no longer there may be afraid of going to sleep in the future in case the remaining parent disappears. A child who has witnessed a terrifying incident may be re-living it in his mind. The main remedy for nightmares is ROCK ROSE as this helps to ease the panic and the terror of the frightening dream. If the child wakes hysterically, then it would also be useful to include CHERRY PLUM to bring calm back to the mind. RESCUE REMEDY is ideal for night terrors and is an excellent remedy to always have on stand-by.

In addition, however, it is vital to consider what might be causing the bad dreams because until the cause is tackled, the dreams are going to continue. A child suffering with recurring nightmares in which unpleasant experiences are re-lived, would benefit from HONEYSUCKLE, and also WALNUT for protection against the disturbing influence. MIMULUS is the remedy for known fear, and would therefore be appropriate in many instances, whenever there is a reason for the anxiety, such as the fear of a parent leaving the home. However, if the basis of the fear is concerned with the *safety* of a parent, RED CHESTNUT would be more applicable as this deals specifically with the type of fear and anxiety related to the well-being of those we love.

| **I** | **FEEDING** | There can be no doubt that the ideal purpose-made baby food is breast milk. Women have |

breasts for the sole biological purpose of producing milk for their babies, just as any other mammal would suckle their young. Breast milk, apart from being cheap, safe, convenient and readily "on-tap", is nutritionally balanced for a human baby with all the correct constituents in the right quantities. So why, if nature has built women to feed their babies, are there some who are unable to? Perhaps it is because human beings have evolved so much intellectually that it interferes with basic in-built mechanisms. Emotionally we are so finely tuned that even slight disturbances can throw hormones out of balance, and because breast feeding relies on hormonal activity, this too can be affected by stress and other emotional upsets. Tiredness, depression, marital strain, worry about other children, to name but a few, can antagonise a smooth and relaxed approach to breast feeding and may indeed play havoc with milk production altogether. Remedies to help relieve the mental negativity that may be causing the "block" will therefore help the mother and her baby to feel more relaxed which is the first step towards success.

Before we move on to some of the other issues and problems concerned with feeding generally, let us consider a few difficulties that may arise immediately before and after the arrival of a new baby, and the remedies that would be appropriate. OLIVE would help relieve the initial tiredness which may stem from sleepless nights in the last few days of pregnancy and during labour, or exhaustion because there are young children in the family to tend to and care for. And let's face it, young children are a handful at the best of times, never mind when a woman is carrying a heavy mature pregnancy and all her energy is needed for the delivery of the new baby. Olive would be helpful before the baby is born if tiredness is a problem, as well as afterwards to aid recuperation and to help replenish lost energy. RED CHESTNUT would help the mother who is afraid for the health of her baby, or over-anxious about the wellbeing of her other children in her absence. PINE would help the mother who feels guilty about not being able to successfully breast feed straight away, feels she has failed and let herself and her baby down. WHITE CHESTNUT would help with persistent worrying thoughts, causing mental arguments and repeated niggles in the back of the mind. GENTIAN would give encouragement to the mother who feels disappointed in herself and depressed, because the close unity and warmth that she imagined would take place during breast feeding is instead a fraught and anxious time. Post natal depression can also cause difficulties for the mother trying to establish a positive feeding routine. MUSTARD is the remedy to help this kind of depression. CHERRY PLUM is also helpful if she should feel the mind beginning to give way, or overcome with desperate panic. Another remedy which is helpful after childbirth is WALNUT. This eases the transition and helps the whole system to settle down. A mother's emotions are soon transmitted to her baby, which usually only serves to make matters worse. If you are struggling to breast-feed and are taking remedies to help you to be more relaxed, then your baby will respond positively and will also benefit from what you are taking because it will be transferred through your milk.

It is not, however, only emotional disturbances that hinder attempts at breast feeding. There are many other obstacles in the way too – attitudes, practicalities, sociability – numerous hurdles and ideas to come to terms with and accept. Breasts are, after all, apart from being milk secreting glands, sexually erotic organs and some women, as well as their male partners, find it difficult to accept that a baby should suckle a breast that has, until then, always been associated with sex. For some people, breast feeding is intolerable for this reason, something that they feel is sexually repugnant. CRAB APPLE would help those who feel that it is unnatural or distasteful, and those who cannot bear the thought or the sensation of a baby feeding from the breast. WATER VIOLET would help the woman who feels that her body is too private to entertain the idea of exposing her breasts, even for her baby; VINE for the woman who feels strongly that she prefers to retain her breasts as primarily sexual organs and therefore stubbornly refuses to even *try* to breast feed. CHICORY and VINE are remedies to bear in mind for your partner if he has this attitude, as these remedies will help him to be less possessive of your body (CHICORY) and less ruthless in his demands (VINE).

WILD ROSE would help the woman who resigns herself to either breast feeding when she *doesn't* want to, or to her apparent inability to feed successfully when really she would like to. GORSE will help the woman who gives up hope of succeeding. CENTAURY is the remedy to help the woman who does not breast feed because she is dominated or feels threatened by the preferences of her partner. For similar reasons, a woman who is "badgered" into breast feeding against her will would also benefit from this remedy.

Sometimes the problem that arises is not so much a dislike of the idea of breast feeding, but rather a disbelief that one's breasts are adequate. Some women find it hard to accept that they could possibly be capable of producing enough milk to satisfy a hungry baby. It is, however, the breast *tissue* that produces the milk, and this has little to do with the overall breast size. What makes breasts big or small depends on the amount of fat they contain, not the milk secreting glands. A woman with small breasts may indeed be taken by surprise when her milk does begin to form, to find that her "flat" chest has expanded into a full and rounded shape, and all of a sudden she is needing a substantially larger bra size!

Society unfortunately has not, until quite recently, made it very easy for nursing mothers. There are many shops which now thankfully have special facilities for changing nappies and feeding, but there are still many which do not, and this, along with the problem of having to manoeuvre a pram in and out of tightly sprung swing doors, buy clothes without being able to first try them on for size, negotiate stairs and escalators in busy stores, or try to comfort a hot and bothered baby in the middle of a supermarket, is really no joke! Finding somewhere suitable to breast feed *as well* may be the last straw!

Another stumbling block is often encountered when a mother needs to return to work soon after her baby is born. Unless her employer has a crèche facility, she may find it impossible to keep up regular breast feeds. It is of course, possible to express the milk so that it can be given by bottle, but this is a cumbersome method to employ full-time, although it does have a number of bonuses – father and grandparents can share the feeding which helps them to feel more involved, and it gives the mother a little more freedom to devote some time to herself and her own needs.

There are, however, some women who, despite their desire to breast feed and persistent attempts, find that they, for one reason or another, simply do not succeed. These women may feel terribly disappointed (GENTIAN), blame themselves (PINE) or feel angry with their "inadequacy" (ROCK WATER). But a woman should never feel guilty for something she has no control over, and just because she has had to turn to bottle feeding, she should not feel or be made to feel that her baby is receiving second rate care. Baby milks these days are as close to breast milk as possible and there are thousands of bottle fed babies just as healthy and content as those who have been breast fed.

Breast feeding is not always easy, and although I would encourage mothers to at least give it a try, it is also important to consider the feelings of all concerned. A calm and relaxed mother will help promote a calm relaxed baby, and so if she finds that she cannot cope with breast feeding, dislikes it too much having given it a reasonable chance, or simply prefers not to, then she must not condemn herself for deciding to bottle feed. A content bottle fed baby is, after all, much better than a distraught breast fed one!

❀ COLIC

There are times, however, no matter how content and satisfied mother and baby are, when for some unknown reason the infant becomes difficult to settle and quieten. Assuming all the usual and likely explanations – wet nappy, thirsty, hot, cold etc. – are eliminated, a baby's fretfulness may be due to colic, a problem which is stressful not only for the baby but the parents too because they feel so helpless at being unable to do anything to help the little one in distress. True colic fortunately is not as common as one might think, because although we often hear complaints of "my baby has colic", it is not always actual infantile colic, but wind or a tummy ache for some other reason. Colic itself follows a familiar pattern, occurring in the early evening. Every evening. It can last up to about three hours and nothing will quieten or calm the baby for long. It may be possible to pacify briefly with a cuddle, suckling or belching, but it does not relieve the situation completely. If your baby has colic-like symptoms but in a haphazard fashion, such as presenting at other times of the day, or only once in a while, then he is not likely to have colic. If your baby's distress *does* conform to a regular pattern however, and it is concluded that colic is the reason, then the general belief is that, unfortunately, there is little you can do other than to accept it and wait for it to pass, and in the meantime give your child all the comfort it needs during these miserable attacks. Nevertheless, it would be advisable to speak to your doctor who will be able to examine your baby if necessary and reassure you that there is nothing physically wrong. Unfortunately no-one really knows why colic should occur and why it should attack some children and not others. If the cause could be identified then a successful treatment could be found. Thankfully, however, colic does not extend beyond about three months and frequently clears up when the baby is old enough to take solids.

Most baby care books will therefore tell you that there is nothing you can do for your baby, but the Bach Remedies can, at the very least, offer a little help to ease the distress. If we consider how *we* feel when we have indigestion, for example, we can appreciate what it must be like for a little baby who does not yet understand what the pain even means. The fear and tension that are so often caused by pain may soon create a vicious circle – the tense mood causing tension in the body which, in turn, makes the pain worse. The Bach Remedies do not treat the colic directly, but they can break into this distressing cycle and help to relieve the fear and anxiety that is responsible for much of the tension. There is nearly always at least an element of shock, terror, panic, agitation and bewilderment in a baby's distress, and many mothers have found RESCUE REMEDY extremely helpful – it can be diluted into a little boiled water and then dropped into the baby's mouth, or if you are breast feeding, wet your nipple with the dilution and allow your baby to take it from you direct, or you can give it in a drink, or on a dummy or by spoon. Alternatively you could dab it onto the baby's forehead, fontanelles, temples and wrists, and if you dilute it in a little warm water, it can be applied to the abdomen too. You may prefer to use the **Rescue Remedy Cream** for this purpose, gently massaging it onto the baby's tummy. If you can at least take the edge off the pain, then you will be doing a great deal to help your baby.

❀ DIMINISHED MILK SUPPLY

Apart from colic, another common reason for a baby being unable to settle after a feed is that the feed itself has not been satisfying. As the day wears on, a mother's milk supply may lessen, and so by the evening, especially if she has had a tiring day, she may find that as the infant grows, she is unable to satisfy him. If tiredness is your problem then OLIVE will help you, although it is also important of course to try and make sure that enough rest is taken and that you are finding enough time to eat properly and drink plenty. These seem very obvious remarks, but when one is rushing around looking after a demanding baby all day, it is very easy to skip meals, bolt your food or leave a meal unfinished, and getting used to cold cups of tea is almost obligatory!

As the baby grows and its digestive system becomes more mature, there will come a time, in any case, when milk alone will not satisfy its hunger. Sometimes it is necessary to supplement breast feeding with a bottle feed at times – this is not uncommon and again, you should not blame yourself or feel inadequate because you cannot cope with the demand. We are all different and whilst some women can go on for months and months efficiently producing milk, there are equally many women who find their breasts "drying up" early. There is no right or wrong; and no woman should be judged on her "performance".

❀ WEANING

Once the baby is about 4 months of age, its digestive system has reached the stage when it can tolerate a semi-solid diet, and the insatiable appetite, screams of hunger and discontent are nature's way of telling you that the time for weaning has arrived.

Weaning is another period of change for your baby. Having been used to milk and suckling from a teat or nipple for the first few months of life, accepting a hard spoon and a completely new type of food may take a lot of getting used to, and at first he may stubbornly reject it. It is, however, important to persevere – gently of course, no need to force feed – because he will have to adapt to this new diet sooner or later. Calm persistence at this stage will work in the end, and it is far better to persevere now than to forget it and try again in a few weeks by which time your baby will be older and wiser and therefore likely to be even more stubborn! WALNUT is a useful remedy to aid the transition and help the baby adapt to a new feeding routine. VINE will help the child who is so strong willed that you end up with a real fight on your hands. IMPATIENS will help the baby who gets irritated and short tempered. BEECH will help the baby who gets annoyed and will not tolerate the spoon in his mouth, struggles to be free or spits the food out again.

At about six months of age, the baby develops a "chewing" reflex and so at this stage it is important to introduce a few soft lumps to the food – mashed rather than puréed – so that the chewing action can mature. If nothing is forthcoming to stimulate this reflex, then it may be lost, making the introduction of mashed food more difficult. Even though the time may be right, however, the baby has to put up with yet another change to its diet and may be reluctant to take it at first. Once again, WALNUT will aid the adjustment as well as other remedies such as those mentioned above, as required.

Whereas some babies are reluctant to eat, and parents are required to rack their brains to dream up a novel way of introducing the food to make it acceptable, there are others who are over-keen. A child who eats more than enough rarely presents a problem, but a child who eats too little provokes endless anxiety. But is that child *really* not eating sufficiently? It is natural for parents to make every effort to ensure that their child is eating "enough", and so it is not surprising that it causes so much worry! It is the toddler and pre-school child who usually present "problems" with regard to eating, but children naturally go through phases of wanting very little food, or hardly eating at all. Forcing them to eat usually only serves to reinforce the "problem", and because stubbornness is also normal, the child will refuse all the more if too much fuss is made. If, however, you are concerned, your family doctor or child care clinic will reassure you.

Sometimes feeding can provide an opportunity to identify your baby's type remedy – not that he necessarily needs a remedy *now*, but if at any time for any reason he or she should be out of sorts, it is always helpful to be able to give a remedy for the character as well as for the mood. Some babies may get in a temper or frustrated and impatient if the spoon is not filled and directed towards their mouth quickly enough. IMPATIENS is the indicated remedy here, and would also be for those babies who are developmentally forward and eager to feed themselves, grabbing the spoon or parent's hand and pulling it towards the mouth. This is, of course, something you will wish to encourage because the child is developing all the time and so has to learn new skills, but if it causes irritation, bad temper or stress for the little one, then the remedy is there to help. VINE and VERVAIN children may also display similar tendencies because they too are astute, alert and quick witted and are often demanding and excitable.

A baby who is entirely placid, who does not seem to dislike *anything*, and accepts without question the parent's authority, may be a CENTAURY baby, or WILD ROSE if there seems to be a "don't mind/don't care" attitude, showing neither enthusiasm nor dislike. CLEMATIS is for the baby who seems to be thinking about something else at feed-time, inattentive and distracted; CRAB APPLE for the baby who eats very "neatly" and looks dismayed at drops of food on its clothing or hands. WATER VIOLET for the baby who is very "ladylike" or "gentleman like" and has a delicate, dignified manner.

In all aspects of life, feeding included, a child's personality will shine through. Physically, we are all basically the same, but are characteristically very individual and have a unique behaviour of our own. It is this individuality, which we see in all the day-to-day activities, that helps us form a complete picture of the child's character and, through that, their personal remedy.

IV | **TEETHING** Teething can begin at any age – and occasionally, babies are born *with* teeth but usually it begins between three and six months. The first teeth to come through are, most commonly, those at the front – either the top two or the bottom two, although usually it is one of the lower teeth that emerges first. The younger the baby when teething begins the easier it is because the gums are softer and so the consequent discomfort is less severe. However, teething is notorious for causing a few problems, although these vary greatly in severity from one baby to another. If your baby is having trouble, you may like to try diluting a few drops of RESCUE REMEDY into a little water and then gently rubbing it onto the baby's gums with your finger.

Impatience, restlessness and bad temper are commonly encountered as a result of pain and irritation. Understandably, a young baby cutting its first few teeth and feeling a discomfort which it doesn't understand, will be similarly agitated. IMPATIENS is an excellent remedy for quelling irritation, and CHERRY PLUM is very helpful for the loss of emotional control. Both remedies are contained in Rescue Remedy which will have a generally calming influence. WALNUT, the remedy for change, is also very useful to remember at this time as teething is another developmental milestone when adjustment is needed.

Other remedies that may be helpful are CHICORY if the baby is clingy and does not like to be left on his own; BEECH for the intolerance of the "horrible" tooth that is causing so much pain; WILLOW if he is miserable and cries constantly for pity; CRAB APPLE as a cleanser – the desire to be "rid" of the aggravating discomfort. It may be helpful to anticipate the whole affair by massaging the baby's gums with Rescue Remedy as suggested above, at intervals before the tooth actually emerges. There are a number of tell-tale signs that will inform you it is about to happen – excessive dribbling, red cheeks, restlessness and crying, baby unsettled and difficult to comfort, chomping on fist, and a hard lump underneath a red gum – although sometimes an intervening factor will give rise to similar symptoms to throw you off the track. It may be helpful to provide something hard on which to chew – teething rings are ideal as they are easy to hold, but a raw carrot, piece of apple or hard crust are far more tasty, and also introduce the baby to new textures and the taste of different foods.

ELIMINATING

What goes in, naturally must come out! Getting rid of waste, therefore, is as natural and essential as eating and drinking. Why then, is so much fuss attached to it? Why do people become obsessed with it, find it funny, embarrassing or disgusting? Perhaps it is the fault of modern society values, because tribal communities accept it as a natural process and do not attach to it the same sort of prim squeamishness as do so called "civilised" communities.

The organs of the body responsible for the formation and release of urine are the kidneys, which filter the blood and remove excess water and soluble waste, and the bladder into which it drains and is stored. There are two tight bands of muscle fibre called sphincters which control the release of urine. The internal sphincter, that which is closest to the neck of the bladder, opens and closes automatically, but the external sphincter is controlled voluntarily. It is this voluntary control that the infant must learn, but until he does, urine voiding is a reflex action and occurs as soon as the bladder reaches a certain capacity.

Voiding of faeces is also a reflex action. As food enters the stomach, the colon automatically contracts, and for a baby, filling the nappy is a reflex response to the food entering and the body's waste passing through the system. On reaching the rectum the nerve endings pick up the sensation of fullness and the anal sphincter opens to release the stool. Conscious control is possible once the feeling of fullness is realised.

The consistency of a baby's stool is something that often causes much anxiety for the parent, worried that it might be too soft, too hard, too frequent or infrequent, the wrong colour, too smelly, or not smelly enough! Breast fed babies tend to have softer and more yellow stools, and may well have a dirty nappy after every feed, although some babies only open their bowels once or twice a week. It is not so much the frequency that is important, but the consistency. Bottle fed babies tend to have paler and more formed stools, although all babies' stools should be generally soft. Green offensive stools may be in response to a digestive upset. Hard stools are an indication that the baby is taking insufficient fluids, something which is not likely to occur in babies who are being breast fed successfully, or in bottle fed babies when the feed consistency is correct. In hot weather, however, it may be necessary to supplement the milk with drinks of boiled water in between feeds. Once solids are introduced to the infant's diet, the stools gradually take on a more adult consistency – and a stronger smell! – and additional liquid may be needed as certain foods have a dehydrating effect. CRAB APPLE, being the cleansing remedy, may be useful should the baby become constipated or suffer a bowel upset.

❀ POTTY TRAINING

Potty training is not likely to be effective until the child shows signs that he is aware of a full bladder or rectum. It is not until about 18 months of age that sphincter control is developed and as the infant becomes sensitive to the bladder filling, the emptying reflex action begins to disappear. Similarly, it is the sensation of fullness of the rectum that helps the infant learn to control defaecation. Because these sensations are immature until about 18 months, there is usually little point in attempting to potty train until then. But all children are different. Some will be ready earlier, others may wait until they are about two years old. However, 18 months as a general guide is about right *usually*, so look out for the signs around that age!

Once again, potty training is another milestone and something else to get used to. WALNUT therefore is the remedy to help make this transitional period easier. Hopefully, it will be a straightforward event, and the child will get used to controlling its bladder and bowels without too much bother. For most children, it will indeed be a smooth and natural process, but sometimes problems do arise.

We generally grow up regarding faeces as "dirty" and do not want to touch them or look at them or smell them for long, but in early childhood, they can be the source of immense fascination. Children who are learning to recognise what the full sensation in their bowels means, soon become curious about the end result. They may begin to delight in it and *want* to look at it and even touch it. This is not being naughty or dirty, it is natural, so although you will want to discourage your child from actually handling his stools, it is something that needs to be done tactfully so that he does not become hurt or frightened. Children can become very attached to their stools and may be upset when they are flushed away. Some children are very proud of what they have "produced" and so indulgent behaviour and desire to show you may emerge. Naturally, you are pleased that your little child is learning to use the potty, so gentle praise is encouraging, but try not to overdo it – recognition of his call to defaecate or empty his bladder is a natural process and so too *much* praise may be confusing rather like someone becoming over-excited when you swallow a mouthful of food – you would probably wonder what all the fuss was about!

❧ SOILING

The fascination with this newly acquired bowel emptying skill may cause a few problems. As already mentioned, flushing the toilet or emptying the potty may upset some children, and if it all grows out of proportion in the young mind, a reluctance to let the faeces go at all may develp, resulting in constipation because the child tries to hold on to them, unwilling to risk them being flushed away again. If it is severe enough, the constipated stool causes a blockage, and then as more faeces build up behind, an "overflow" occurs, causing a dribbling of watery excrement which is difficult to control and thus results in constant soiling. This problem usually occurs in older children, rather than the 2 or 3 year olds and is not generally common. However, "accidental" soiling is very common in the younger age group, and so should not necessarily be interpreted as a behavioural problem or abnormality. It is rare for older children to soil, but for those who do, the constipation issue needs to be investigated and most importantly, the reasons *why* it is occurring.

Children learn not only through their own experience, but also through observation, the example set by parents and other closely related adults. If the mother (for example) has a hang-up about toilet habits, perhaps feels disgusted herself about the very thought of defaecation, then this may, unintentionally, be conveyed to the child who in turn also develops a form of neurosis about going to the toilet. If left to grow and develop into adulthood, this "disgust" of faeces, defaecation, urine and urination may lead to a belief that all genito-anal functions are dirty and this may result in persistent constipation or even sexual problems. It is therefore clearly im-portant to tackle the difficulty at an early age and resolve it before any of these more severe problems develop. Before we move on to the remedies to help children directly, let us turn our attention to those which can help *in*directly, by assisting parents with difficulties they too may be facing.

One of the hardest things for a parent to acknowledge is that their child's problem may be an echo of their own problem. If you *do* have a problem yourself there is no use ignoring it. That will not help yourself or your child. However, there is one thing you should always remember, and that is, whatever the problem might be you should not burden yourself with guilt. It is not your fault, any more than your child's problem is *his* fault. You were a child once and so the difficulties you face now most probably had their roots in your own childhood and you would therefore have had little control over what was happening. Facing it and acknowledging it is nothing to be ashamed of, and although you may regret it and not want to talk about it, just think how much better and how relieved you would feel if you could be rid of it altogether. The first step is that important self-acknowledgement, and then the desire to help yourself. Once this first big hurdle has been overcome, the next stage will follow naturally. The remedies are there to help, and any one or a combination may be required, depending on your own individual needs. Some remedies are commonly required because they are indicated for just this type of problem, so I will describe them here:

FOR CLEANSING – CRAB APPLE This remedy is for anyone who feels a certain amount of disgust at bodily functions, and this might include vomit, phlegm, semen, vaginal discharge as well as urine and faeces. It is also for anyone who dislikes themselves, considers themselves worthless, dirty or vile; for anyone who hates the sight of themselves and thinks they have an ugly face or body. It is also the remedy for those who, because of their outlook, feel the need to repeatedly wash their hands or even their whole body over and over again, unable to bear to touch anything that may be remotely dirty. For those who develop an obsession with cleanliness and become overly house proud, Crab Apple is indicated, in whatever degree it might be apparent. The Crab Apple remedy, taken for any of the above categories, in part or in total, will have a cleansing effect upon the mind and thus help to remove the idea of contamination, so that the sufferer realises there is really nothing to get so worked up about, that a little dust will not hurt them, and that emptying the bladder or bowels is as natural a part of life and living as eating, sleeping or breathing.

FOR FEAR – MIMULUS This is for any associated known fear, for example, being afraid that going to the toilet will be painful, or afraid that you may pass blood. This would be a common fear and wholly understandable if blood *has* actually been passed, in which case medical advice should always be sought. Mimulus however, helps to ease the fear that may be standing in the way of your management of a normal daily routine.

FOR OBSESSIVENESS – HEATHER For those who, like the Crab Apple, are obsessed with their trouble, but instead of shying away from it, hating it and being disgusted by it as the Crab Apple person would, this remedy is for those who revel in it, *want* to talk about it, and disclose intimate details that the listener may not really want to hear! The positive side of the Heather character is that of a person who enjoys company and likes to talk. They are therefore very friendly people, good company and generally fun to have around. When something bothers them, however, their thoughts dwell on the particular issue and their conversation begins to revolve around it. The Heather remedy helps to divert the self-obsessed thoughts so that the "problem" gradually becomes less significant.

FOR PRIDE – WATER VIOLET This is for those who, unlike Heather people who *need* and *want* to talk, avoid the subject, pretend it is not there, and would *never* divulge their feelings to a stranger. It is far too personal and nobody's business but their own. It is something they feel they must cope with and deal with alone, far too embarrassed to go to anyone for help or advice. Water Violet folk are naturally private and very personal people. They give little of their true feelings away and do not express their emotions in public. They are dignified and refined people, gentle and quiet, and truly a blessing to have around, but they can be their own worst enemy and battle on alone with a problem which could otherwise be dealt with and treated, simply because they cannot bring themselves to discuss it. Self help is therefore often the Water Violet's first (and sometimes only) avenue, and if they can read about themselves in the privacy of their own home and their own mind, then it will be a relief to discover their own personal remedy which can assist them. It is there to help them drop the shield that is kept so firmly in place around them, not so they lose their gentle dignified pride and privacy, but so they can feel more comfortable reaching out for help and not be embarrassed to ask.

Children may have similar traits to those described above, and so similar remedies would apply to them too. If for example your child was revolted at the thought of passing a stool, or was disgusted, ashamed or distressed at having soiled, wet or made a mess, then

CRAB APPLE would be the appropriate remedy. Similarly traits of the WATER VIOLET may be noticed, in which case this remedy would be appropriate to a child of this nature too. The Water Violet child would be likely to hide his soiled pants, too embarrassed to show you or admit what had happened. He will not like to be watched when he goes to the toilet or sits on the potty, and if he is, this in itself may be enough to make him retain his stool or even his urine.

Fear is also a common element in children – MIMULUS is the remedy to help general known fears, but sometimes the fear does not have a definite cause, and is rather a sense of apprehensive uneasiness, a feeling of fear without really knowing why. If you ask the child what he is afraid of, he would say something like "I don't know, I'm just scared". ASPEN is the remedy to ease this frightening and eerie apprehension. Sometimes, a child might *say* he does not know what he is afraid of, and so it remains hidden and causes turmoil inside the little mind. On the outside the child may appear to be calm and undisturbed which is sometimes a false sense of security for the parent, although with young children who have not really mastered the art of completely disguising their feelings, parents invariably notice that "something" is wrong, even though the child will not admit to anything. AGRIMONY children are usually out-going and happy, but do have this tendency to hide what is on their mind. The Agrimony remedy helps them to share it which is the first step towards solving the problem.

Children who feel threatened by other children or dominant teachers, relatives or siblings, would be helped with CENTAURY. Children who do not want to "waste" time by attending to a call of nature would benefit from IMPATIENS. Children who are so engrossed in what they are doing that they "forget" to go to the toilet, would be helped with VERVAIN. Those who feel a great sense of loss, terribly upset at seeing their excrement being flushed away would benefit from STAR OF BETHLEHEM, the soothing remedy, and GENTIAN for those who become despondent about it. Those who worry, perhaps with disturbed and restless nights, would be helped with WHITE CHESTNUT which calms turbulent thoughts. Those who stubbornly refuse to use the potty or toilet, perhaps in an act of rebellion – those with a very strong-willed character who are difficult to restrain because they know their own mind and precisely what they want – would benefit from the remedy VINE. This would help to ease the aggression and desire to fight everything, so that a more relaxed attitude has a chance to develop.

Conversely you may have a child who is totally blasé about it all – a "shrugged shoulders" approach. For this child, WILD ROSE would be appropriate. Or for the absent minded, dreamy child who does not always seem to be aware of what is going on, CLEMATIS would apply.

As always, every child is different and so each one needs to be assessed on his or her own individual merits, and remedies chosen according to individual needs and personality. There is no single remedy or specific mixture for soiling – each child will have a different reason, a different personality and feel differently towards it, so what is right for one child may not be right for another. The remedy is not therefore for the presenting problem directly, but for the underlying cause which ultimately lies in the individuality of the child concerned.

❀ BED WETTING

Occasionally, bed-wetting is due to a urinary tract infection, but mostly it is either due to sleeping very heavily or to stress. The occasional accident is quite normal and is common during illness, especially when there is a fever, high temperature or delirium. Sometimes a dream may cause the bed-wetting – dreaming of being on a toilet for example – and in such a case, the child usually wakes up shocked to find a wet bed. It can be extremely upsetting, even if it is something that has happened only the once, for some unexplained reason, and especially for the older child or young teenager who would understandably feel terribly embarrassed about the whole episode.

Practical help, such as avoiding drinks directly before bed-time, may be needed to help these children, but the remedies can be of great benefit, particularly for those children who are disturbed by stress, or for those who feel utterly dismayed at what has happened. Once again it is necessary to consider the child's overall personality and temperament in order to select the most appropriate remedy.

CRAB APPLE would help the embarrassment and sense of shame or disgust; CLEMATIS the heavy sleeper who is also drowsy and dreamy during the daytime, and AGRIMONY would help the child who has something on his mind but keeps it all to himself, pretending nothing is wrong. These children may try to hide their wet bed – the young child covering it up with the bed-clothes and hoping no-one will notice; the older child perhaps trying to dry the sheet or attempting to wash it himself, panicking in case he is found out. CENTAURY is for the child who is upset by bullying or the aggressive behaviour of children at school, and who continues to worry at night. MIMULUS is for the child who may have been previously reprimanded and is afraid of being told off again. ROCK ROSE is for the child who is terrified of something – perhaps nightmares causing a loss of control during sleep. CHERRY PLUM would be helpful in this respect too as it is the remedy to calm a runaway mind. Both remedies are included in RESCUE REMEDY which would be generally calming for agitated restlessness in the night. The child for whom bed-wetting has become a habit, or who does not seem to learn from experience and thus fails to correct the pattern would benefit from CHESTNUT BUD. WALNUT, being the remedy to ease transition and break habits, would also be helpful.

There are times when a child might bed-wet, soil or smear for attention. If this is the case, CHICORY will help the child learn to be independent and not demand so much of other people's time and attention. Chicory children have a great need for love and comfort, and may become clingy. There may, however, in addition to this need for the closeness and company of a parent, be an under-lying fear – perhaps afraid of being left alone, fear of the dark, intruders, spiders etc. – and the child tries to overcome this fear by demanding or manipulating attention. MIMULUS, ROCK ROSE or perhaps ASPEN would help to ease the frightening thoughts, WHITE CHESTNUT for the persistent troublesome thoughts, and CHERRY PLUM, ROCK ROSE or RESCUE REMEDY would help to stabilise an imagination that has caused panic in the young mind.

Whatever the reasons, there is usually little to be gained by reprimanding the child for wetting the bed because there is, more than likely, some external stress that is ultimately responsible, and the child is therefore not necessarily doing it deliberately. By getting to the root cause, and by looking into what may be troubling your child, which may involve approaching the school or even examining a relationship problem or other upset within the family, the right remedies can be chosen to help all involved.

❧ ❧

Parents naturally are often concerned about giving their child "medication" for straightforward aspects of normal healthy childhood. It may be difficult to accept a remedy for a problem without also having to concede that there is an inherent behavioural or psychological condition that requires treatment. After all, getting frustrated when feeding or potty training is not an illness – all children get annoyed or irritable, become demanding or selfish from time to time – but sometimes these normal human emotions stand in the way of a child's progress, and then what should be straightforward milestones *do* become traumatic and problematic. The important and reassuring thing to remember about the Bach Remedies is that they assist rather than correct, and give a helping hand rather than remove one's own autonomy. You are not therefore giving your child a suppressant or a crutch, but essentially part of life, and because the remedies are part of the Life Force itself which surrounds us all and is indeed part of us all, they are as helpful to little children as they are to adults. Used to achieve their full potential, they are remedies for the entire family – mum, dad, children, grandma, grandpa – even the pet rabbit!

CHAPTER 3

A Child's Social Development

DURING EARLY CHILDHOOD, an enormous amount of growth and development takes place over a short period of time, and it is therefore a constant period of change and learning. There are routines to get used to and experience to be gained through play, interaction and relationships within the family. Gradually the child learns social skills and socially acceptable behaviour. It is through exploration, trial and error, first hand experience and imitating the example of others that these skills are accumulated and shaped in keeping with the child's innate and individual personality.

PLAY

As the child begins to think and organise his thoughts, play and environmental stimulation is very important. At around 12–18 months, the child is at the age of exploratory behaviour and so he needs toys that are interesting to handle, those that make noises, are of different shapes, colours and so on. Plastic shapes that he has to "post" through matching slots on the lid of a container would be an ideal toy for a child of this age.

Although speech is still developing and only a few words are decipherable, the child will be understanding much more than one might think, and so repeating colours, explaining, calling items by their names etc., will help the child learn what they are, even before he can actually pronounce the words. Children enter into spontaneous play because they are inquisitive and want to explore. For example, if a toy or interesting object is placed on the floor, the child will experiment with it and find out by trial and error what it will do, learning all the time. If the task proves too difficult, then he will be irritated by it and quickly lose interest, but if it is appropriate for the developmental age of the child, it will hold the attention and keep him amused for a long time, and give him a sense of achievement at the end.

There are two types of play – active and passive. Babies and young children are mostly involved in active play – playing games, running, climbing and so on – whereas in older children, adolescence and teenage years, play goes through a more passive phase – watching television, reading comics and magazines or books for example. Environmental factors can affect the type of play in which a child will indulge, and because children mimic parents and older siblings, they will often follow similar pursuits. If the parents watch television for leisure, read a lot or listen to music, their children will be likely to adopt similarly passive play. On the other hand, if the parents are active sports-people or enjoy walking, cycling and other similar activities, then it is likely that their children will also take an interest in sport and enjoy active play.

Play itself has several functions. Physically it develops muscles and helps coordination. It can be therapeutic as it releases tension, and despite the agitation children may express when they cannot do something, play acts as an outlet for frustration. It is also educational as it encourages the child to explore and motivates him to learn and develop perception. As a child plays with other children, he will begin to compare himself with them and then start to learn about his own strengths and limitations. It is a means of learning and developing social skills by the interaction that is necessary during play with someone else – whether it be an adult or another child. It is also creative and helps the child's imagination to develop.

The development of spontaneous play goes through several stages, beginning in early babyhood, when it helps to develop motor skills and movement. Then, at about three months, when the child begins to really handle things, he learns about coordination between hands and eyes, and oral exploration – the "everything-in-the-mouth" stage. Then comes imitative play, at round 7 months, when the child watches and tries to copy – begins to hold his bottle, tries to feed himself, and attempts to comb his hair for example. By about 18 months, the child will be engaging in constructive play, acting out a pretend situation as a game, and announcing out loud what he is doing. Language is also developing, echoing what is heard and thus building up a vocabulary, all of which helps the child's perceptual and social development. Soon the child learns to sustain play for longer periods, and by about 4 years, games which involve rules are enjoyed – "hide and seek" for example. Later, as the child gets older, there is the development of recreational interest or hobbies, and of course this type of play extends right into adulthood – building models, board games, stamp collecting, fishing, painting etc. – although adults do not usually refer to, or admit that by indulging such interests, they are in fact "playing"!

Young children – 18 months–2 years – tend to play by themselves, learning to share games and toys a little later. At this age they are becoming quite imaginative and from about 2 years the child begins to indulge in fantasy play. This is the beginning of hypothetical thought – a transition from "let's pretend" to "what if". CLEMATIS children are naturally creative and so they may be noticed at this age to be particularly imaginative, and become totally "lost" in their fantasy games. Imaginary friends are very common, especially for children with no brothers or sisters, or those who are constantly fighting with siblings. It is also said that intelligent children tend to invent friends.

The greatest expression of creativity is through drawing. At first, when a child is given a pencil or crayon, it is usually held in the fist and the drawing is just a series of dots as the child stubs the crayon on the paper. He does not really know or understand what he is doing at this stage, but soon realises that the crayon he is holding is actually making those marks. As with anything else, he will then begin to experiment and explore its possibilities and very soon his artistic talents will have progressed to lines and then scribbles. He will also learn how to hold a pencil correctly – in fact children do this automatically as part of their natural development, although it may be a little clumsy at first. As the child learns to draw circles etc., he encourages himself by describing what he has drawn. Gradually, from about 3 or 4 years, these drawings will start to resemble more accurately what they are meant to be. From about the age of 8, the child will begin to draw what he actually sees, and once he can draw something he really likes – a train, an aeroplane or the family dog for example – then he will draw it all the time. Paints bring out a new dimension, and although they are messy for young children, are an excellent way of developing creativity from about 3 years onwards. Let the child make a mess – he will learn that way – but make sure you have plenty of large plastic sheets and aprons handy!

All children are different and yet they will follow a similar pattern of development. Drawings are similar, the content is similar etc. – i.e. when drawing a house, it usually has four windows, one in each corner, and a door in the middle. If the sky is painted, it will be a blue strip at the top of the page with a big yellow sun and the obligatory rays... But even so, each child is drawing his own picture and so there is a mark of uniqueness about each one – an expression of individuality.

A child's emotional outlook can be observed through his paintings – a child with something on his mind may present aggressive pictures, or draw something or someone damaged in a particular way if that person or thing has upset the child. For example, he may draw people with sad faces if the child sees unhappiness around him, or may block out the faces of people he dislikes as a way of pretending they do not exist.

If you feel your child is disturbed by something, brought to your attention by his behaviour or through his drawing, the remedies can be of great help, but it is important to ask two questions – "why?" and "how?" Why is he disturbed? How is it affecting him? How and why does he react to it? Quite often children will not express these emotions in any other way, and if it were not for their pictures, we may never become aware that anything is wrong.

AGRIMONY children hide their fears and anxieties – they would be the children to keep a disturbance concealed, their only outlet perhaps being their drawing and painting. CENTAURY children may also hide the way they feel. These particular children are timid and find it hard to stand up for themselves, become down-trodden and dominated by the strength of others. They may harbour feelings that they dare not express, and suppress them instead, so they fester in the little mind all the same, and like the Agrimony child, feelings can find an outlet through creative work. A child who has an unpleasant memory that preys on his mind – perhaps he has witnessed something violent or has lost a parent, grandparent, brother or sister – may find an outlet for his grief through art and may draw people who are dead or maimed. HONEYSUCKLE is the remedy to help these children release the unpleasant memory from their mind – to help them understand and let it go. STAR OF BETHLEHEM would help ease the shock and sorrow, and WALNUT would be a helpful remedy if the child has been unsettled by an upheaval.

In aspects of play generally, traits for which the remedies are indicated will be expressed. Once again, however, it does not mean that a child necessarily needs a remedy because he fits a particular description – that is simply his personality – but these guiding factors and observation of how he behaves will help you to choose remedies accurately if and when the child *does* need them. For example, the child who seeks reassurance and needs to be praised because he is uncertain that he has done something correctly, and constantly asks "is this right mummy?", "will you show me again how to do it?", is displaying traits of CERATO and the remedy would help this child to believe and be convinced of the correctness of his own actions and desires, and help him to know and have faith in his own mind. The child who is undecided about any given choice and spends much time pondering, perhaps unable to choose which toy to play with, would need SCLERANTHUS to make him more decisive. The child who is totally disinterested and shows little enthusiasm may be a WILD ROSE child, or HORNBEAM if weariness or lethargy is apparent. The child who becomes discouraged if he is unable to complete a puzzle or draw a certain picture, or cannot put something together properly, would benefit from GENTIAN as this remedy would give encouragement and help to lift the despondency. Children who are easily bored with games or toys, impatient to move on; whose concentration span is very limited – often bright children who need much stimulation and seem to have endless energy – may well be IMPATIENS children, and the remedy would help them have more patience and be less hasty. CLEMATIS, on the other hand, would help those who become bored and *disinterested,* lack concentration or daydream. VERVAIN would help the enthusiastic child who becomes frustrated. VINE would help the child who plays aggressively, and CRAB APPLE would be for the child who is extraordinarily tidy, making sure toys are always put away neatly. ROCK WATER children may also be like this – they are perfectionists and like to set an example to a younger sibling, as well as for their own benefit because they like to feel pleased with themselves. HOLLY will help the child who seems to get angry or in a temper with toys; perhaps spitefully mutilating a doll or breaking something because he does not like it. CHERRY PLUM will help the child who loses control, throws things, rants and raves, gets in an uncontrollable temper and becomes hysterical.

❧ ☙

When it comes to making ones own entertainment, children take the lead. Give a small child a cardboard box and he will make it into a boat, car, train – anything he wants. Children frequently get far more enjoyment out of an everyday item that has cost nothing than from an expensive toy. They have such a vivid imagination that play, games and fun come naturally.

Children also go through phases of enjoying a certain *type* of play or particular game, and similar games are shared by children all over the world – skipping, playing "chase", "it" or "tag", hopscotch, swapping beads, marbles or stamps are just a few examples, and now video and computer games have almost become as commonplace as a television set in some homes. Pocket sized versions make them even more manageable, and many children carry these mini-games around with them and play them at every possible opportunity!

Children become immersed in what they do, but becoming entranced by a video game can have repercussions. Some games vividly portray violence by characters being beaten, shot, knifed, blown up, set alight etc., and because the child is not simply watching but actively involved in the shooting, stabbing, fighting or bombing, it becomes all the more realistic. "Virtual reality" games are even more life-like, and children can become completely drawn into an imaginary world to the exclusion of the real one.

This does not necessarily mean that video or computer games are dangerous. They can be educational as well as recreational but "video addiction" is, for some children, a real phenomenon. "Every-thing in moderation" therefore is a sound motto, and if other hobbies are pursued as well, they will retain a distinction between what is real life and what is not. It may sound ridiculous to think that a child can confuse computer graphics with actual reality, but to children, *life* is a game, and because their imagination is so powerful, the two may easily become intermingled, possibly resulting in some unfortunate consequences.

Not all children who play with these games, of course, are in need of remedies, but for those who are, here is a selection that may be particularly helpful: WALNUT to break the link with the habit and offer protection from the compelling influence; CLEMATIS to bring reality back into focus; VERVAIN to relieve the tension and over-excitement that causes the child to become fixed and obsessed; CHERRY PLUM to help them gain more control over their thoughts; CRAB APPLE to help cleanse the mind of its obsessive involvement; VINE to overcome the desire to dominate others; HOLLY for a desire to injure, kill or torture; IMPATIENS to help them control their excitement and to channel it positively and constructively with greater patience.

| TEMPER | As children grow and develop, they are learning all the time. They see activities going on and they |

want to try to do things themselves and so learn how to dress themselves, feed themselves, do up their shoe-laces, wash the dishes and so on, and by so doing, gradually become more independent. Very young children are astute mentally before they become physically proficient, and so although they *want* to do something are not always mature enough to accomplish it. This leads to a great deal of frustration, and the resulting tantrum might be interpreted as bad behaviour although it is perfectly normal for a child to express his frustration in this way.

When a child gets annoyed with his inability to do something, or with someone else for not letting him, a common reaction is temper. Some children have other ways of expressing their anger and frustration – head banging (see also Chapter Two) or breath-holding for example – but whatever the reaction might be, it is upsetting for both the child and the parents who find themselves unable to do anything to either control or settle their young child. Temper tantrums usually reach their peak at about two years, hence the term "terrible twos", but they can begin much earlier than this, making potty training and other disciplines extremely trying at times, and may extend until the child is about three. The tantrum is not due to badness but exasperation at his own limitations. He tries to communicate but is not always understood because although he knows what he *wants* to say, cannot actually express himself verbally in comprehensible language. This is also the age when the "negative stage" begins, when the reply to any request is "no"! Much of the time, young children are eager to help and *enjoy* doing things, but sometimes there is stubbornness mingled with this willingness which is, essentially, a test of how far they can stretch your patience. If asked to put something away, they will refuse. If asked to be quiet, they will make more noise. If an attempt is made to get a child to eat, he will push the spoon away, turn his head and close his mouth tightly. If asked to "come here" he will move further away....

This period of young childhood is packed to capacity with an enormous amount of input, and understandably these things are difficult to cope with all at once. A number of remedies are indicated to help children come to terms with this particularly frustrating period of growth. IMPATIENS for the impatience they have with themselves, their toys, situations, their parents etc; when things are not happening quickly enough or when they feel they are tripping over what they are trying to do or say. Children of this age are also quite active and get over-excited. They like to shout and make themselves heard and so may be constantly noisy as a result! If this is causing problems for the child, Impatiens would help to ease excessive excitability, and thus relieve the tension. VERVAIN would also help, especially if the child is "highly strung" and difficult to calm down. An inquisitive child who is eager to learn, enthusiastic about everything, always on the go, never sitting still, may be a Vervain *type*, and predisposed to this kind of frustrated tension.

BEECH is for intolerance, and so is another useful remedy at this time. For example, when the child cannot get his shoe on – intolerance of his own clumsiness and lack of skill, intolerance when you try to comfort him or show him how it should be done. VINE would help the strong-minded child who likes to dominate and gets in a temper when he cannot have his own way – "I want, I want". For those who "want it *now*", IMPATIENS would be indicated. CHICORY would help the child who becomes annoyed in a selfish manner – "It's mine, it's mine" – and has a tantrum in order to get it!

Sometimes the child will become rigid with frustration, having been out-witted and thus annoyed with himself at not being able to do something properly. This rigidity and desire for perfection would be helped with the remedy ROCK WATER. For the child who sulks when something does not go according to plan, or if reprimanded, WILLOW is the remedy needed to promote a more positive frame of mind. For the child whose frustration is so great that he shows signs of self destruction or obsessive behaviour, CRAB APPLE would be helpful, along with ROCK WATER for the self-punishment, denial and demands the child places upon himself. HOLLY would also prove helpful for the anger, spiteful behaviour or temper towards siblings or parents. CHERRY PLUM would help ease the temper that gets out of control.

Once again, it is important from your point of view, to remember and be reassured by the fact that your child's temper tantrums do not necessarily mean he is in need of psychiatric help. For the majority of children, these displays of temper and "odd" behaviour are the result of frustration, and therefore part of normal healthy development.

LANGUAGE AND INTERACTION

First of all, we might ask what is language? Is it speech or is it communication? We can communicate without saying any words, and we can speak without communicating anything. The *object* of language however, is to communicate. How it is achieved, therefore, really does not matter. Sign language is just as communicative and meaningful to the deaf as spoken language is to those with normal hearing, and so words are just another tool of communication.

We also acquire language in order to interpret ideas and organise mental processes. When we think, we are effectively talking to ourselves. The mental images are transferred into the language we know in order to connect those thoughts. Children tend to think in words, and this is demonstrated by the way they talk through what they are doing, drawing or playing. As we get older, we are able to interpret mental images and think in terms of pictures – remembering places, road signs or faces for example, and by using a form of photographic memory, we might try to "read" from what we remember of a book, recipe or newspaper article. Having seen it once, we can recall it to a certain extent in our mind and then examine it in an attempt to glean the necessary information. Some people are much better at this than others, but we are all capable to a limited degree.

Communication, language and speech development all begin very early in babyhood. The new-born baby communicates by crying, but as he gets older, he begins to communicate through smiles, babbles and body language. Hands are very important language tools for young children as they will show you what they want by pointing, holding something out to you, reaching for the spoon to inform you that they want to feed themselves, and so on. This form of communication is enhanced verbally as the child learns to speak. A child goes through a developmental speech pattern, able to make different sounds at different stages, beginning with "ba", "da", "ma" at about six months, and "mama", "dada", "baba" at about nine months, and speaking two or three recognisable words by about 15 months or so. The baby understands what is said to him long before he can say the words himself. Listening, processing what is heard and vocalising a response, even though the vocalisation is not recognisable language, nevertheless means that the child is clearly communicating. *He* knows what he is trying to say, even though it might sound like incomprehensible gobbledygook. Parents tend to understand and are able to translate the babble which helps the child develop his communication skills.

The object of language is to communicate with other people, and for most of us this is done through speech. It is not only the words we say that form the communication, but the way we say them, the emphasis we place on certain words, our facial expression and the intonation in the voice are all ways of giving what we say greater meaning. The acquisition of language therefore is an important part of the child's social development and needs to be encouraged.

Interaction is ultimately what language is designed to achieve. However, being able to communicate does not necessarily mean that our interaction with others is comfortable. Our personality plays an important part in our ability to interact successfully. Shyness for example (see VIII) can get in the way of approaching others, joining in a conversation or contributing to a discussion (MIMULUS).

A dominant nature may conversely present a threat to others, frighten them and, as a result, interaction is hampered (VINE). Impatience (IMPATIENS) and intolerance (BEECH) may also be anti-interactive.

When we meet someone new, we tend to instantly form an opinion, and even if we try not to, we cannot help our first reaction. Some people we meet seem so confident and sure of themselves that we might feel in awe of them. On the other hand, that seemingly confident person may not be like that at all, but merely putting on a front to cover up for what they believe is a weakness (AGRIMONY or ROCK WATER). An overpowering, strong and dominant person (VINE) may find gentle timid people (CENTAURY), irritatingly placid, whereas the gentle person may find the strength of certain people overwhelming. There are also the unexplained phenomena that figure in how we interact with other people. Just "something" about a certain person attracts us to them, or repels us; makes us feel comfortable or uncomfortable in their presence. Children tend, on the whole, to be more open in friendships. They have not had the restrictive influences imposed upon them that adults accumulate during their lives, and so young children generally by-pass the "first impression" stage and simply accept others for what they are.

Somewhere along the line, during maturity, we seem to lose that innocent acceptance and as a result, cut ourselves off from many would-be or could-be friendships. The roots of this transitionary change seem to occur during our school years. During this time we are exposed to new rules, new people, a complete menu of ideas and expressions, and we spend virtually *all* our growing years at school, so it is bound to have an effect on us and influence the way we develop quite considerably.

GOING TO SCHOOL

The first taste of school may be nursery, or a pre-school play-group. At nursery, the child has the opportunity to get used to being with other children, to play with different toys, develop social skills by eating with others at set meal-times, get into a routine and, of course, broaden and practise communication; language, speech and interaction. The child also learns how to stand up for himself, experience being hurt by other children, how to comfort and how to share. The list of benefits is endless. I cannot think of many disadvantages, providing the nursery school is reliable, with an adequate number of staff to make it safe and provide all the children with enough individual as well as group attention. Every child is different of course, and so it is necessary to consider the child's individual needs, but on the whole, nursery schools provide an ideal bridge between familiar home life and the demands of full-time education.

When a child first goes to school, he may feel unsettled, may not like it and may not want to leave you. He may even run away from school. WALNUT will help the child to settle and adapt to a new routine and adjust to his new surroundings and people with whom he spends his day. If the child is nervous or afraid, MIMULUS would help him feel more secure, or ASPEN if his fear is vague and non-specific. CHICORY will help the child who does not want to leave you, clings, and cries and screams in an attempt to stop you leaving the school gates.

Going to school not only means the child has to get used to a new set of values, discipline and a new routine, but also signals the end of infancy and the beginning of childhood. He learns how to handle other children, how to respond to them, how to manipulate ideas and so on. With this new awakening, comes independence. The child realises that he can do things by himself and will *want* to do things by himself. Although it can be a little sad for a parent to see the baby in their child disappear forever, the establishment of independence and the development of his personality and social skills need your support now more than ever before, and so naturally it is important to encourage your child in what he does; take an interest in what he brings home from school, and feel proud of your budding artist, creative writer or developing mathematician!

| **V** | **BEHAVIOUR & ACHIEVEMENT** |

Frustration has a lot to answer for when it comes to difficult behaviour in childhood. This is partly due to the expectations in achievement demanded of children as they grow up because, as some psychologists argue, there is a shift from a system at home which is essentially "person centred" (when children are praised for *who* they are), to a system at school which is "achievement centred" (when children are praised for what they can *do)*.

Fulfilment of a child's true capacity for learning, understanding and creating is linked, to a large extent, with the response he receives when he first learns something new. For example, if a group of children are shown a picture of a parrot, and asked what it is, one child might say "a picture", and no matter how genuine that child might be in the conviction of his answer, may receive the reaction "don't be stupid". Another child might say "a bird" which may be rewarded with a half-smile informing the child that his answer was good, but not good enough. The child who says "a parrot", however, receives applause and praise. Children who receive negative feedback repeatedly will become frustrated and lose interest, and eventually this will have a negative effect on their potential to learn. Similarly, those who are bored because they are given dull and insufficiently challenging things to do may also respond negatively, become confused, and despite their fear of failure, in effect, *learn* to fail.

There are also those children who find an outside interest that they *are* good at, but because the interest is too obscure and not catered for by the school, they may not have the chance to develop their new found interest or talent, resulting in disappointment, dejection and an even greater sense of failure. It may even lead to rebellion, disruption, learning difficulties or some other behaviour which is essentially an active expression of frustration.

As a result, some children seem to go out of their way to be cheeky, destructive or disobedient, and those who are not receiving the attention they need (or want), may adopt other ways to obtain it – refusing to eat for example, or to go to sleep, deliberately telling lies, stealing, bullying, injuring themselves etc. At school, a child may get attention by shouting, getting over-excited or being disruptive. There are numerous devices employed by children to gain adult attention, but the most important question as far as the Bach Remedies is concerned is "why?". Is the disruptive, rebellious behaviour masking something far deeper, something that is the true problem? Usually it is, and in order to help the child, it is essential to find the "real little person" underneath the brash exterior – the true personality. It may be that the disruptive behaviour is part of his basic nature. He may be a very strong-willed child who likes to get his own way and misbehaves when he cannot have it. This child would need VINE for the aggression and perhaps CHICORY for the selfishness. The child who is deliberately attention seeking, clinging, using tactics such as crying, feigning illness or "nagging" to get his own way, would need CHICORY to encourage him to be more independent and not so possessive.

Other remedies that would be helpful are GENTIAN for discouragement; WILLOW for self-pity or resentment because of the lack of interest shown in him; GORSE for the child who is pessimistic, gives up hope and stops trying; ELM for the child who feels overwhelmed with the responsibility of having to live up to certain expectations; PINE for the child who feels guilty because he has not achieved or reached the appointed standard; ROCK WATER for the child who reprimands and punishes himself because he has not come up to scratch; SCLERANTHUS for the child who is undecided about the correct answer – is it this or is it that? – hesitates and may therefore miss the opportunity to get it right at all; CERATO for the child who needs and seeks confirmation and reassurance, and SWEET CHESTNUT for the child who is desperately trying to get it right, and who sinks deeper and deeper into a sense of despair if his repeated attempts fail.

Some children *do* know the answers and will always proudly stand up and give the correct reply. If the teacher presents the class with a difficult question, these children will always be the ones who hold up their hand, or explain to the rest of the class when several wrong replies have been given. They have the confidence to make their understanding known, and although they often genuinely want to share that understanding, they are frequently referred to as "know-alls", "teacher's pets" or the "swots" of the class. Being called names and constantly sneered at can soon lead these children to withdraw into a shell. Although they are *naturally* confident, they may feel uncertain, and so would need LARCH to restore their confidence once again. Other children really do not care what others think. They bravely stand up to adversity and do not let anything get them down. They are OAK types. Those who appear to be a little superior, adopt an attitude that sets them apart from and above the rest, would be the WATER VIOLET types and this remedy would help if that aloofness caused them to feel lonely or alienated.

To overcome embarrassment, many children are apt to deliberately make a fool of themselves, encouraged by the laughter of their class-mates, and may "show-off" to detract attention from their ignorance or overcome their uncertainty and insecurity. If they can make the others laugh, they will be liked, and if they are liked, they feel more confident and comfortable. This kind of mask that hides an inner whirlpool of emotion would be helped with AGRIMONY. LARCH would also help the underlying lack of confidence, and SCLERANTHUS and/or CERATO, the lack of certainty.

It may be, however, that the undesirable behaviour is due to an underlying fear – afraid of not being noticed; afraid of being ignored; afraid of not having any friends. Children suffering like this may be harbouring a lack of confidence, no belief in themselves or what they are capable of, in which case LARCH would be helpful. This remedy would also help those who are afraid of failure, but for children who are afraid of the repercussions of failing – fearful of the reaction and disappointment of parents and teachers – would need MIMULUS. Those who put on a boisterous façade to mask their fear of failure, of being reprimanded or of speaking out of turn would be helped with AGRIMONY, an important, helpful and comforting remedy on such occasions, coupled with the remedy or remedies that are in keeping with the child's manifesting behaviour.

If we look at "disruption" in another light, the "disruptive" child may simply be enthusiastic. He might be a bright child, bored by the pace at which he has to learn, and would actually benefit from being in a more advanced class. The child who "shows off" by shouting answers in class, therefore, may not necessarily be seeking attention or praise, but simply bursting with enthusiasm because he genuinely knows. Naturally, one would not want to quash that thirst for knowledge but should the enthusiasm cause frustration, a child of this nature would be helped with VERVAIN. IMPATIENS would help the child who is impatient to reach the conclusion of the lesson, or cannot wait for play-time, and thus sits and fidgets, in an attempt to find something to relieve his boredom. The Impatiens child's attention span is limited, and he may resort to annoying the pupil in the next seat, writing on the desk, making paper planes and sending them flying across the room when the teacher is not looking, making a noise with his chair as he wriggles around in it, or interrupting with comments or questions that are totally unrelated to the topic being taught.

| VI | **DYSLEXIA** |

Dyslexia is a particularly distressing learning difficulty. It is when letters and/or sounds become muddled, and dyslexic children see words and misinterpret them by reading backwards, or seeing certain letters in reverse. Seeing a "p" as a "d" or "b" for example, or reading a word like "dog" as "god". Sometimes multiples of words are read in reverse order "turn right" as "right turn". Writing may be affected; the child finding it very difficult to spell words correctly and write letters in the right order. Speech too may be involved, with mispronunciation of words, either pronouncing them backwards or omitting letters as though perhaps the whole word sound had not been heard – "feet" instead of "fleet" or "bake" instead of "break".

Dyslexia has been greatly misunderstood and children have been accused of being lazy, disobedient or stupid. This is not of course the case and although there are *some* children who may use their disability to gain attention, or occasionally having noticed the attention a sibling or friend receives as a result of being dyslexic, attempt to copy them in order to receive similar attention, dyslexic children do not acquire reading, writing or speech difficulties deliberately. On the contrary, they may have above normal intelligence but are held back if their condition is not understood properly and are therefore not given the appropriate learning opportunities or educational aids that would enable them to reach their full intellectual potential.

It is only natural for parents to be concerned and worry in case their child will never be able to read or write properly and thus face insurmountable problems in later life. Whilst parents need to be active in the child's stimulation and help by obtaining the appropriate assistance for the child's individual needs, dyslexia in young children is not something that is necessarily going to present lasting problems or interfere with the quality of life. Sometimes it represents only a mild hiccup in the child's language development.

For more severe forms of dyslexia, there are a number of methods employed to correct the misreading and writing. However, one of the biggest problem areas for children who are dyslexic is coping with the lack of understanding that surrounds them and the consequent ridicule that may come their way from other children at school. Constant remarks of "look here stupid" and "you're thick – you can't write properly" are bound to have an effect on these children who may eventually believe that they *are* stupid if they are subject to remarks like this for long enough. A lot of encouragement and reassurance is therefore vital to help them deal with the thoughtlessness of other children – sometimes the thoughtlessness of some adults too. This is really where the Bach Remedies can be of help, gently coaxing back the child's belief in himself, restoring lost confidence and repairing a damaged ego. LARCH would help the return of confidence; GENTIAN gives encouragement, and CERATO helps to reassure the ego. Some children may develop a guilt complex, believing that it must be their fault, and thus constantly apologising for doing or saying it "wrong". PINE would help such a child. ROCK WATER would help the child who reprimands himself, or puts himself under undue pressure, forcing himself to achieve. This is of course not necessarily a bad thing, but if it should cause suffering and mental rigidity, then the Rock Water remedy simply helps the child to be more relaxed in his approach; MIMULUS would be the remedy for the child who is afraid or shy; WATER VIOLET is the remedy for children who cut themselves off and lead separate and lonely lives; CLEMATIS would help the child who drifts into a world of daydreams or lacks concentration; IMPATIENS would help the child who gets irritated by his shortcoming, or who gets into a temper because he is slow.

Again it should be emphasised that a certain amount of apparent dyslexia in young children is quite normal and an accepted part of language development, but if it continues, it does need attention to avoid more serious difficulties in later life, and hopefully will have been anticipated and corrective measures put into action before that time arrives.

VII | **BULLYING** | Bullying at school can be a difficult problem to deal with. It affects not only the bully and the bullied but the parents, the teachers, the rest of the class, maybe even the entire school. The repercussions and wider involvement can be far reaching.

The one who is the primary target – the child being "picked on" – bears the brunt of the bully's spite or threats. The bullied child, therefore, needs help and reassurance, comfort and support, but it is often this child who denies that anyone is causing any trouble and refuses to talk about it even when parents, having noticed a change in the child's mood, suspect something is wrong. Perhaps these children are afraid of their parents' reaction, or the consequential hassle of an angry father (for example) making a "scene" at school. Or perhaps these children do not want to appear weak or unable to fight their own battles.

There are many different reasons why a child might keep it all to himself, but in order to assist with the remedies we need to know the answer, and ultimately the best person to provide the answer is the child himself. This may require a lot of patience and gentle coaxing and it may be necessary to invite the child to talk to some-one else – an older sister or brother, an aunt, uncle or grand-parent for example. The child may feel more comfortable if he is able to talk to someone to whom he is not immediately answerable. We can however, *imagine* what the child is going through, and sense, at least to a certain extent, the mood of the child and how this differs from his normal mood. The child may seem pre-occupied, depressed or frightened. He may have a frightened look in his eyes; may make up a variety of excuses as to why he cannot go to school. He may even make up a fictitious reason and attach the blame to something else, such as not having done his homework, or feeling ill. Most people will be able to recall an occasion when they have felt so frightened or nervous about a forthcoming event, that a feeling of nausea and maybe actual vomiting has occurred, and so a similar reaction may occur in a child who is worried about facing an uncomfortable situation at school.

The remedies can certainly help but it is important to establish how individual children react in order to select the most appropriate remedies. Not all children will react to being bullied in the same way. Some will accept it, resign themselves to it, not *bother* to fight back, and instead, just put up with it. These children would need WILD ROSE to help them take more of an active interest in what is happening and to give them the motivation to face and deal with the situation. The child who is afraid, whether it is of being hurt, of the repercussions and consequences, or feeling afraid of being frightened, would need MIMULUS. There may however, in addition to these known fears be an undercurrent of unexplainable apprehension – a sense of "something" being about to happen... For this type of fear, ASPEN is the remedy required. ROCK ROSE would also be an important remedy to consider. It is for terror or panic, whenever the fear is greater than the "everyday" nervousness of Mimulus, generating much stronger emotions. Rock Rose is one of the ingredients of RESCUE REMEDY which also contains **Star of Bethlehem** for the shock of the first encounter with the bully, and **Cherry Plum** for the panic that stems from imagining all sorts of terrible scenarios, so Rescue Remedy would be a helpful remedy to give in an emergency – if the child becomes very distressed before going to school, for example.

If the child cannot stand up to threats and meekly submits to the bully's demands, then this not only inflates the bully's ego, but also saddens the child who, by virtue of his very nature, finds he has dug a hole for himself from which he cannot escape. The remedy for this type of child is CENTAURY. It is for those of a gentle, kind but submissive personality who are easily dominated and cannot say "no" to anyone. They can, however, become their own worst enemy because their gentleness does not provide them with the "hardness" they need to deal with the situation. The Centaury remedy helps these children to realise that they will not be hurting anyone by saying "no", least of all the bully, and having done so, they will feel proud of themselves because they *have* been able to stand up to the aggression and not allowed it to get the better of them. Then, next time, if there is a next time, they will know that they have done it before and can do it again. WHITE CHESTNUT would be a "helper" remedy for worrying thoughts that go round in the mind, causing the child to have disturbed nights. WALNUT will help protect these children from outside influences and thus help them to remain detached and not so drawn into the bullying tactics. CHESTNUT

BUD would be appropriate if the child *does* manage to stand up to the bully but then falls back into the same situation time and again. SWEET CHESTNUT would help children who feel desolate, trapped and unable to see a way out.

SCLERANTHUS would help the child who hesitates about either what to do or whether or not to tell someone, first deciding on one approach and then changing his mind. CERATO would help the child who does not have enough belief in himself and therefore doubts the correctness of any decision he might make. LARCH would help the child who does not have sufficient confidence to speak out or confront the bully, and MIMULUS would help the child find the courage to carry it through. Children who struggle on against adversity, withstand parents' willingness to make a complaint, and instead insist that they must deal with it themselves and fight their own battles, would benefit from OAK to help them maintain or recapture their natural strength. The true Oak will win in the end!

The bully, on the other hand, is the dominant child, overpowering others who are "weaker". One would associate this aggressive behaviour with VINE. Indeed this may be just the remedy that the child needs because the *negative* side of Vine is certainly aggressive, demanding, intimidating and sometimes cruel. Vine therefore is a very important remedy to bear in mind. In addition to this, however, HOLLY is the remedy for spite, desire for revenge, hatred, jealousy etc., all of which can result in taking aggressive action. There may be a bitter grudge being harboured – perhaps the bullying child believes that he has suffered some misfortune that is the fault of the other child – and so bullies by way of satisfying that resentment. WILLOW would help to rid the child of this bitterness, and help him to forgive and forget.

In some cases the aggression may only be superficial, and underneath it all there may be a very insecure child or one who feels unwanted, unloved and deprived of attention. He therefore turns this inside out to gain the attention and control that he so desperately wants, and by taking such a forceful position he tries to get noticed and earn respect. If this is the case then we need to help the child come to terms with his insecurity and help him not to feel so isolated.

❧ ❧

We all have something to contribute to life, in our own way, and it does not matter whether we are quiet or outspoken, for the role we play will use whatever talents we possess. It is, however, difficult for most children to appreciate this because they have not usually had the experience in life to have developed an understanding of the differences in human nature, or the plight some people have to live through. BEECH would help the child who is critical and intolerant of other people's downfalls, finding it hard to understand why they do something in a way which to them (the Beech), seems stupid, irrelevant or incompetent. IMPATIENS would help the child who is irritated by what he considers to be the slowness of other children, and sometimes Beech and Impatiens are indicated together – impatience and intolerance running in parallel. HOLLY would help children who are spiteful towards the shy, timid child in the school.

SHYNESS

Shyness is something that is experienced by most children at some time. When taken to see someone they do not know, or when a person they have not met before comes to visit, it is quite usual for a small child to "go shy". But this usually lasts only a short while and once he has got used to the unfamiliar person, soon resumes his normal talkativeness and behaviour. For some children, however, shyness is more than a momentary disposition but something more fundamental and, to these children's despair, often follows them throughout their growing years. Some people go into adulthood without ever having shaken it off. For these people, shyness is part of their nature. The Bach Remedy to help is MIMULUS which tackles the underlying nervousness, fear and timidity that are ultimately giving rise to the shyness. Nervousness at meeting new people, fear of having to talk in front of a group, anxiety at the thought of entering a room of strangers and so on, are all aspects of the Mimulus person's nature. If an adult is shy, they most likely will have experienced similar shyness during childhood, and anyone who is familiar with these feelings will probably nod in agreement when I say it is one of the hardest things to cope with – in adulthood as well as childhood. Truly it can be desperately uncomfortable, particularly for a child who has to cope with ridicule from other children when he gets tongue-tied, stutters or does not seem to have anything to say. In fact, these children may have *plenty* to say, but because they feel so nervous and uncomfortable in a situation where they are expected to speak out, anything they might have wanted to contribute to a conversation evaporates, the mind just goes blank and their embarrassment causes them to stammer (see also IX). This happens in adulthood too, and it is being under pressure that makes a person of this nature unable to focus their thoughts on what they want to say.

It is difficult for any child who is trying to make friends, to fit into a new school where friendships amongst the other children have already been established, but for a shy child, it is particularly difficult to settle in and really feel accepted. Children often lack the understanding and compassion that develops later in life and so can be thoughtless and collectively (albeit usually unintentionally) cruel in their attitude. A child who stands out from the crowd because he does not make friends easily, may soon become the object of fun. Whispering when the child goes past, name calling, unkind remarks and ostracism are just some of the painful experiences some children have to endure and learn how to cope with. It is hard, and although Mimulus is the remedy to help them *gain* courage, without realising it they are, in fact, demonstrating a *great deal* of courage through their endurance, and so sometimes both negative and positive aspects of the remedy may be apparent together. Mimulus will, however, help children of this particular disposition feel less nervous, more able to approach other children, have the courage to speak out and find the words that would otherwise escape them. Their basic nature will remain intact, and so although they may always be inclined towards shyness, with the help of their remedy, they will be able to cope with it so that it no longer stands in the way of their enjoyment of life.

LARCH would also be a helpful remedy for this type of child as often the nervousness and timidity are coupled with a lack of confidence, and if this is the case the two remedies would work together to help the child gain more confidence in him/herself, and overcome the nervousness and fear.

BLUSHING

No child wants to appear foolish in front of his school-friends, but the classroom offers the ideal opportunity to show himself up! Feeling ridiculous, saying something that is "stupid", or not knowing the answer to an apparently simple question can shatter confidence into tiny fragments. Standing up alone, whether it be to confess that one does *not* know, or even to recite a correct and well-rehearsed answer is acutely embarrassing. Blushing is a response to this embarrassment, and is one of the worst aspects of shyness. If a shy child is picked out in class to answer a question or demonstrate something in front of the other children, blushing is almost conditional – shyness and blushing seem to come as a package! – but no matter how much he *expects* to blush, it is no easier to bear. It is a give-away sign to everyone else – a blatant announcement stating "this child is embarrassed; this child is shy". The child tries so hard to conceal it or stifle it, but there it is – a red face for everyone to see, and *feeling* the colour rising just makes it worse. The child feels even more self-conscious, and the blush becomes even deeper. It is like a nightmare. There is often an attempt to hide it by declining the head, allowing the hair to drop over the face as a form of camouflage, holding the hands up to rest on the cheeks, hoping that no-one will notice, and the thread of dignity that is grasped by these attempts may be all that is preventing the inevitable blank-mindedness. The worst thing that anyone can say to a person who is blushing is "oh, you've gone all red"! Especially when it is in front of others and followed by splutters of laughter! Anyone who has experienced such appalling moments in childhood will acknowledge the feelings described here. It is not something one easily forgets, and can indeed make school-days the worst days of one's life instead of the best. It is so sad that a child should be subjected to so much unhappiness, and often loneliness, just because he is quieter than the other children. Fortunately he is not likely to be the *only* child in the school – it is quite a common problem and so once settled, friends *are* established which makes life much easier.

We have discussed Mimulus and Larch as remedies to help in this kind of situation, but there are others too that might be indicated. A child who is quiet, gentle and kind-hearted, would be suggestive of CENTAURY. Children who hide how they really feel – those who try to hide their shyness firmly behind outward gregariousness – would need AGRIMONY. If a child is covering up a definite shyness or fearful nervousness in this way, then both Agrimony *and* Mimulus would be indicated. Similarly if a child was trying to cope with a desperate lack of confidence by trying hard not to *appear* that way, Agrimony and Larch would be a suitable combination, and WHITE CHESTNUT would help to ease the mental torment.

Some children may become very pessimistic, or resent the remarks. If a child should become depressed, then remedies that give him encouragement and lift his spirits are required. GENTIAN would help him come to terms with a set-back or disappointment. GORSE would help the child who gives up trying, and as a result, may give up on school-work, or may not want to go to school any-more. WILLOW would help the resentful child or the one who sulks and feels sorry for himself, dwelling on his misfortune – "why have I got to be like this? What have I done to deserve this affliction?" – and falling into a negative downward spiral becoming withdrawn and unable to think about anything other than his own difficulties. Willow would help children who feel this way to direct their thoughts outward; help them feel optimistic enough to climb out of the negative cycle of thoughts and think more positively about how to tackle the problem – or even just how to *accept* it and come to terms with the way they are.

IX STAMMERING

This is a common speech problem. It is due to the involuntary repetition or loss of sounds during speech, and the prolongation of certain syllables. In very young children, stuttering or stammering is quite normal and most children will go through a period of tripping over their words. A child who becomes excited, for example may stutter in his attempt to tell you all about it, so the fact that a young child begins stuttering does not necessarily mean that he is going to have speech problems thereafter.

There is often a family history which may suggest that the problem is genetic in some cases, but the fact that parent and child both stammer does not in itself mean that the child has inherited the problem from the parent – he may simply be imitating the parent's speech as all children do when they are learning to talk. Stammering is, however, accepted as being associated with some form of stress. Whether stress is actually the primary cause or simply a contributory factor, exacerbating a problem that is already there, is a wide question, but as far as the Bach Remedies are concerned, it really does not matter. Cause or contributor, it is the relief of the stress which is the key to relieving the stammering. Occasions when the child is relaxed, feels at ease and inconspicuous – when in familiar company such as talking to animals or to a kindly aunt – tend to be stammer-free, whereas situations that cause pressure such as being asked a direct question in the class-room or having to meet and talk to a stranger, or a person with whom the child does not feel comfortable or may be afraid, are when the stammering becomes obvious.

Of course, not all children who are subject to stress will stammer. It all depends on the individual child – some will be affected, others will not. It is the child's reaction to the stress, something that is inherent in his basic personality, that is responsible for whether or not he becomes a stammerer. Children who stammer are often nervous, self-conscious and shy, and there are certain remedies that would help this fundamental anxiousness at the root of the child's inability to cope with stressful situations. MIMULUS would be for the child who is of a shy, nervous disposition. Being the remedy for the relief of fear, it will help such children to have more courage to deal with situations that would otherwise worry or frighten them, and because it is the remedy to help relieve the effects of shyness, it helps them feel more at ease when confronted by groups of people or unfamiliar faces. LARCH is a remedy which often accompanies Mimulus, for it is the remedy to help the self-conscious child recover his confidence. WALNUT would help too because it is the remedy that protects from outside influences and thus will help the child withstand the pressures imposed through the prejudices or opinions of others. AGRIMONY is another remedy that may often be appropriate because it is for those who hide their feelings and try to put on a brave, cheerful and confident appearance. The strain of attempting to cover up their shyness, fear or anxiety, causes the stammering which, naturally, draws attention to the fact that perhaps the child is *not* as confident as he is trying to make people believe. The child senses this and in his attempts to hide the stammering as well as his anxiety, the stammering gets worse. It is a vicious circle, but Agrimony will help to relieve the tension, and thus help the child to be more relaxed which in turn will ease the stuttering.

For some children, stammering is due to an *eager* mind, speed of thought and trying to get the words out too quickly. The vocal chords, tongue and mouth have difficulty keeping up, so the child stumbles over what he is trying to say in his anxiousness to process thoughts into words. IMPATIENS would be helpful in this case because it is for those who are quick minded and have a tendency to talk rapidly. The Impatiens remedy helps to relax the feelings of urgency and thus allows time for the words to form. VERVAIN children are also eager and excitable, and they too may find that in their enthusiasm to say what they think, their mind becomes tense and the connection between what they want to say and what they actually *can* or *do* say becomes muddled and mis-directed.

Stress may stem from an upheaval or distress in some aspect of the child's personal life – perhaps a change has taken place in his schooling, or home-life, or maybe he feels he is under pressure to do well, to achieve and live up to expectations. Children who, for example, are constantly reprimanded for "sloppy" speech, may develop a complex and become so concerned that it deteriorates into stammering. Children who are adversely affected by the discipline and high standards of achievement that their parents, grand-parents or teachers might hold, would be helped with ROCK WATER.

Another element of stammering is hesitancy, indecisiveness and self-doubt. SCLERANTHUS is the remedy to help any form of instability when there is vacillation between one thing and another. If the mind is undecided, then the speech can be similarly disrupted, and Scleranthus can be a very helpful remedy in this respect. CERATO would also help should the child doubt himself or seek reassurance, and once again, LARCH would help the child who has little confidence in himself. There may indeed be an element of each of these states, in which case a mixture of all three may be required.

If the stammering persists, then it would be advisable for the child to receive professional help from a speech therapist who will be able to help the child re-train his speech patterns. The remedies to deal with the causes of the problem in the first place will naturally help this process along, but sometimes physical re-training is necessary as well. Of course, the earlier this is done the better, preferably before the child starts school. Whilst it is advisable to discreetly monitor the child's speech, parents can help by not paying *too* much direct attention to the stammering, and by resisting the temptation to constantly correct. Patience, reassurance and support, with the Remedies as an additional helping hand, are often all that is required for the child to relax enough to forget his difficulty and talk more fluently.

TICS Tics or twitching are involuntary movements such as constant blinking, stretching the mouth, shrugging the shoulder, rolling the head, sniffing and coughing. They are related to some sort of nervousness, worry or inconsistency in the child's life, and may also be brought on by fear or apprehension. In some cases there may be a genetic factor, but otherwise they are usually emotional in origin. There may be nothing in particular that one can put the finger on that might be the cause or the trigger, yet a curious tic of one sort or another develops, sometimes only apparent when the child is totally absorbed in what he or she is doing – drawing a detailed picture or making an intricate model for example. Often the child does not realise what he is doing and even when it is pointed out to him, does not seem able to control it. It is probably best not to draw attention to it as this may simply make the problem worse by provoking self-consciousness and enforcing the idea that the child is "odd" in some way.

The treatment should be aimed at correcting whatever it is that is *causing* it in the first place. For example, if the child is concerned because there is a conflict at home, the tic will usually disappear of its own accord once harmony is restored. It may, however, if it goes on for long enough, become a habit in itself, so that even when the cause of the child's insecurity is corrected, the tic as a habit continues. As far as the Bach Remedies are concerned, it is important to not only establish the cause, but to put it into context with his personality and temperament generally. Nervous children, for example, are likely to respond anxiously to conflict. MIMULUS therefore may be a key remedy for a lot of children, being the remedy for fear and nervousness of anything known. ASPEN, the remedy for unknown fears, is also an important remedy and may, in some cases, be more appropriate than Mimulus (although they can be given together if necessary). Aspen helps the anxiety and feeling of apprehension that may clutter a child's thoughts even when there is no clear reason for the anxiousness. WHITE CHESTNUT will help the child who is worried by an event – starting a new school, or coping with arguments at home or between friends. All children are sensitive to influence but some seem to be more vulnerable than others. CENTAURY children for example are quiet and timid, kind, gentle children who find it difficult to stand up for themselves. Children of this nature, are likely to feel unhappy and ill at ease with any sort of conflict. AGRIMONY children do not like argument either and will try to avoid distress at all costs. Agrimony people pretend that they are happy because they do not want to make a fuss. Children frequently hide their true feelings, in particular when there is a worrying conflict in the home when their security is threatened, and because they may not fully understand what is happening, become afraid, but, they try to stifle their worries. So although one might sense that there is something wrong, the child will be reluctant to divulge what is really on his mind. The inner turmoil that this creates is exactly what Agrimony is for, and is therefore an important and very helpful remedy in many cases. WALNUT is the remedy to protect from outside influences and so it will help to protect the child who has a disturbed home life or difficulty at school. It is also the link-breaking remedy and so would be useful in the breaking of habits. VERVAIN would help the child who is "highly strung", lively and "bursting" with excitement. IMPATIENS would also help the tense child whose thoughts race ahead, and this sort of mental impatience can easily lead to irritation, resulting in the involuntary twitching. ASPEN would help the sense of excitement for no particular reason as this too can cause tics, repetitive swallowing or anxious breathing to take place.

LARCH would help the child who feels self-conscious or lacks confidence. SCLERANTHUS would help the insecure, indecisive child, who may have fluctuating moods. CHESTNUT BUD would help the child who has overcome a tic once, but finds it keeps return-ing. Chestnut Bud is the remedy to help the child learn from his experiences so that he does not follow the same pattern or drop into the same pit-falls.

Sometimes involuntary twitching may occur as a result of tired-ness, in which case OLIVE would be an appropriate remedy. Whereas some children are not aware that they "tic", others are almost comforted by it, and feel they *have* to stretch their mouth or rotate their head (for example) to satisfy this urge. Nail biting is similarly something that many children do as a form of comforter but it becomes a compulsive habit which is very difficult to break. This obsessive pattern would be helped with CRAB APPLE which has a cleansing action on the mind, and WALNUT to break the habit.

A shock or bereavement may equally be the cause of a child's tic. STAR OF BETHLEHEM helps to relieve shock as well as sorrow and thus is a great comforting remedy for those who have suffered dis-tress. The resulting tic, however, may not begin straight away – it may suddenly start some time later, but Star of Bethlehem would still be appropriate for the relief of the shock no matter how long ago the actual event took place. Sometimes children who lose a parent, especially the eldest child of the family, feel responsible for the other children and for the remaining parent, and although some children cope admirably in such a position, others may feel overwhelmed with their new responsible role in life and inadequate or unable to cope with it. If they feel under pressure then they may develop a stress related tic. ELM is the remedy for children who feel this way, and its action is to restore confidence in their ability to cope so they may, if necessary, calmly seek to relieve the burden by asking for appropriate help and support.

HYPERACTIVITY

This seems to be a rather curious label, because who or what establishes how active a normal person should be? What is "normal", and is something that is deemed to be over-active actually *ab*normal?

Many children are labelled as being hyperactive when in actual fact they are only displaying normal childhood antics. Elderly grandparents who have become used to a peaceful, evenly paced life may consider a young child who seems to have an insatiable appetite for activity and whose energy never seems to expire, to be hyperactive. Yet a young mother with two active children of her own, may consider the same child to be lethargic. Hyperactivity, therefore, may be a rather subjective diagnosis. However, there is an established problem area which encompasses children who are, by *anyone's* standards, over-active. They are children who run about all the time, who are *extremely* excitable, jump up and down on furniture incessantly, shout and talk loudly and constantly, and who may also display unacceptable behaviour – breaking, chewing, or destroying things, for example – in their quest to satisfy their boundless energy and excitability. Lying, cheating and inappropriate hysterical laughter are also symptoms of what is indisputably a hyperactive child.

A number of things have been thought to be the cause. Artificial additives – preservatives, colourings, flavours etc. – have all been blamed for hyperactivity in children, and allergic reactions have also been found to occur as a result of eating certain foods as well as the additives they contain. Treatment therefore may include the elimination of possible foods, drinks and certain ingredients patiently and systematically, one by one, until the real culprit is revealed. If this is found to be the cause of the hyperactivity, once it is identified and removed from the child's diet, a marked improvement will take place. Treatment of the cause is therefore essential if the child is to recover his or her normal composure and temperament. There is little use in only providing palliative measures or artificially suppressing the child. This does not solve anything, least of all the child's hyperactivity. However, the remedies, although they may be thought of in the case of allergy-related hyperactivity as a means of only temporarily quelling the immediacy of the problem, or as a passive treatment for the *effect* rather than the cause, can nevertheless be of great assistance, providing the causal factor is also removed. WALNUT can be a very helpful remedy during this transitional period because a child who has become dependent on a food additive for example, may have withdrawal symptoms which are, proportionally, not unlike those encountered by a person who is being weaned off an addictive drug. Walnut helps to break the link.

There are, however, apart from the children whose hyperactivity is physical or material in origin, those who suffer with hyperactivity as a result of emotional instability, and of course with these particular children, the remedies really do come into their own. Symptomatically, remedies such as IMPATIENS for the great speed at which these children move, VERVAIN for the tension, eagerness and excitement, and CHERRY PLUM for hysterical behaviour and loss of control, are all remedies that seem to be most commonly required. Other remedies such as VINE for children who are extremely demanding, aggressive and forceful, and HOLLY for children who display spiteful, hateful or jealous behaviour, are also often indicated.

Certain other conditions sometimes give rise to hyperactive behaviour, and so similar remedies would apply, adapted to suit the individual child's needs.

Naturally, parents are going to be affected by the hyperactivity of the child and may become utterly worn out as a result. Remedies can therefore help them too: IMPATIENS should you become irritable or impatient – perhaps with other members of your family besides the child in question; BEECH if you feel aggravated and annoyed, find it hard to tolerate the child or the situation; WILLOW if you feel resentful about having to put up with such difficulties (a natural response and nothing to feel ashamed about); CHERRY PLUM if you should feel your own mind giving way under the strain; SWEET CHESTNUT if you feel desperate, at your wits end; WHITE CHESTNUT for the worrying thoughts and mental arguments that are most likely going round and round in your mind, keeping you awake at night and tormenting you all day; RED CHESTNUT for natural parental anxiety over your child's well-being, and last, but by no means least, OLIVE for the utter exhaustion!

CHAPTER 4

Family Relationships

ALTHOUGH CHILDREN ARE INDIVIDUAL PEOPLE and have a life of their own for which they will eventually be responsible – making their own decisions, coping with their own disasters and enjoying their own pleasures – during childhood, their lives centre around their family. People bring children into the world, feed them, clothe them, cuddle them when they fall down, look after them when they are ill, but children do not really *belong* to their parents. They are only theirs to protect temporarily because one day they will have to look after themselves, and so it is important, no matter how hard it might be, to let them be independent when the time comes. It is, however, up to parents to provide an environment for the little souls they have brought into the world to live safely and, we hope, happily and healthily, thus assisting them on their journey.

In order to travel through life in the way we hope they will, certain basic needs have to be met – physical care and protection, stimulation and teaching, affection and approval, consistent and appropriate discipline or control, and the opportunity and en-couragement to gradually become autonomous. If these basic needs are not fulfilled, then a piece or pieces of the jigsaw will be missing, and the child's development, especially his emotional development, will not be complete. Sometimes however, this is unavoidable due to circumstances of life, so it is impossible to protect children from everything. We cannot foresee what might lie ahead to turn our world and all our intentions upside down, and whilst *some* children may be deprived of these basic needs due to thoughtlessness or care-lessness, sometimes there are things over which we have no control, so parents should not feel guilty if they are merely victims of circumstance.

However, in order to help children come out on top, it is important to understand what might go wrong and why they happen to behave in the way they do. Let us therefore, examine some of the situations that *can* arise, and their effect upon the children within the family concerned. (See also chapters 2 & 3 for specific behavioural problems).

A NEW ARRIVAL The average nuclear family consists of two parents and the classic "2.4" children. It means that, for most, a second baby will be born at some stage. For the parents this is (usually) an occasion much looked forward to. It is exciting, and will mean a complete family. For the first born child however, it may be a completely different story…

Some children adapt extremely well and the two siblings get on together with little or no jealousy or resentment between them. For others, however, the arrival of a new brother or sister may not be so easy to accept and may herald the beginning of a very emotionally turbulent period.

At the beginning, mum's pregnancy is interesting, something different, and a new member of the family may seem fun at first, but once the child realises that the baby is there to stay, a lot of negative emotions can quickly rise to the surface. Jealousy, resentment, the employment of various attention seeking devices, tantrums… I'm sure there are many mothers and fathers who will be only too familiar with these reactions. It may help to ease the impact if you are able to introduce the child to the idea gradually – get him involved in what is happening and invite him to help with the care of the baby, so that he or she does not feel left out. However, even with the best intentions and well thought out plans, children have a habit of not reacting as we would expect! The remedies, of course, can help to make it a little easier by controlling the torrent of emotions that are affecting the child concerned. HOLLY is the remedy to choose for the jealousy; VINE for aggression and stubborn disobedience; WILLOW for the sulky behaviour due to resentment towards the sibling, or towards you as a parent for (seemingly) ignoring him, and CHICORY for feeling left out and wanting more attention. These three remedies are frequently called upon during this time. Another remedy which is helpful to give is WALNUT because it is for change and so will help the child to adapt to the new family life routine. In addition, consider the way your child behaves normally, at other times, with other things; consider his or her personality and usual temperament and give a remedy that describes this individuality.

When a second baby is born into any family, it is common for the first child to feel left out. Very young children do not fully understand the significance of what it means, and sometimes, even when you may be consciously trying to take as much notice of your first-born as you can, and are fully aware of his or her feelings, it is just a practical fact of life that you cannot give your undivided attention to two children at the same time. If your new baby is unsettled, then it is understandably going to be even harder, and sharing your time evenly is difficult at the best of times! The remedy for a mother who feels overwhelmed with the responsibility, and feels she cannot cope with it, is ELM.

Some children may be afraid of the new baby or afraid of being sent away, of not being wanted or loved anymore. MIMULUS is the remedy to help children who suffer with this type of fear. Quite often, however, the child will just feel "uneasy" – apprehensive about the baby but not really knowing why. This type of fear would be helped with the remedy ASPEN.

Some children may be spiteful towards the new baby – pinching, poking and hitting it. HOLLY is the remedy for this, although it may be associated with fear in which case a suitable fear remedy would be needed as well. Some children, however, do not fully appreciate that the baby in the cot in the corner that looks so much like a doll, is actually *not* a doll! They will then play with it and treat it as another toy – one that works without clockwork or batteries! – and so apparently unkind behaviour, in this case, would be un-intentional.

Whilst there are some children who object to the arrival of the new baby and react with spite, jealousy or disturbing attention seeking behaviour, there are many other children who become highly protective of the baby, look after it, care for it, "mother" it. This is CHICORY behaviour – over-care and concern. Most parents will be thankful that their child has accepted the new baby so lovingly, and this is the positive aspect of the Chicory nature. The remedy would help if the child became possessive. CENTAURY children also have a natural instinct to care. They are not selfish, but will be gentle and genuinely concerned for the baby's welfare, keeping watch to make sure that he comes to no harm, reporting every whimper. They will take great care if they should hold it, and may be nervous of doing so for very long. Children of this placid nature may be afraid of hurting the baby and become over anxious about its well-being, panicking in case something is seriously wrong if it should cry. RED CHESTNUT would be helpful for this type of concern.

The arrival of a new baby may cause uncertainty and as a result, questions about where babies come from may soon follow. It is inevitable that they will be raised one day and the subject often causes parents much apprehension as they wonder how best to explain the facts of life. The day may come much sooner than expected, at an age when one would not think the child old enough to understand, and this is why children at one time, were told that babies were found under gooseberry bushes or delivered by storks... However, if a child, even a very young child, understands enough to query where a baby has come from, then he must surely have sufficient understanding to absorb at least a simplified version of the truth. Naturally, one would not wish to go into explicit detail at this stage, but explaining that the baby grows inside mummy's tummy is often enough to satisfy the curiosity for the time being. However, once that idea has had a chance to be absorbed and formatted in the child's mind, the next inevitable questions will be "how did it get in?" and "how did it get out?" These questions, from the parents' angle, may be a little trickier to answer! Inquisitive little minds always ask "why" and "how", so it is probably a good idea to set some time aside to gently answer the child's questions in a way he will under-stand, tactfully and carefully so as not to instil fear. If there is an opportunity to observe animals giving birth to their young – baby lambs, puppies or kittens – this would be a way of gently introducing and explaining the subject. It may also help, in readiness, to let your child feel your pregnant abdomen, listen to the baby's heartbeat, feel it move and so on. This way, he will get the chance to really understand and feel involved in the whole event.

II | **SIBLING RIVALRY** Although sibling rivalry is generally associated with adolescence (considered in detail in the latter part of the book), a certain amount of rivalry may develop between younger children as they grow up together; each one competing for attention, each wanting to be the most highly praised and regarded. This may lead to a lot of spitefulness, selfishness and provocative behaviour such as telling tales so the other gets the blame for a mishap, or deliberately causing an accident – spilling the milk or breaking the best china – and then once again attaching the blame to an unfortunate sibling. It has even been known for two children to develop simultaneous illnesses as they compete for the "number one" position. CHICORY will help to relieve the selfishness, and HOLLY the jealousy and spitefulness. CENTAURY would help the one who finds it hard to fight back, and WALNUT for them both to get used to, and learn to live with, each other!

Rivalry may also occur with regard to toys, clothes and, when they are older, boy/girlfriends. Again, jealousy rears its head and in an attempt to retain a peaceful and harmonious atmosphere, you may find you have to buy each one the same sort of toys, clothes etc. However, children also have to learn to share, and they may need to share the same bedroom as well as the same toy box. Although this can be good fun at times, it may also provoke arguments, especially as the children get older. With the help of the remedies, however, it is hoped that there will be more fun than unpleasantness, so that they grow up to be good friends in the end.

III | **PARENTAL DISHARMONY** Sadly this is a very common problem, and whilst not all turbulent relationships break down completely, there are plenty that go through periods of separation or some other stormy episode. A child whose parents have endless rows and is therefore subjected indirectly to disharmony within the home, is bound to be upset by it. After all, his home is his world and his parents are those who keep it all together. If he sees or senses that his security is threatened, then he is likely to be afraid, worried or withdrawn. Many children in this situation keep their feelings to themselves and are reluctant to talk about what is on their minds. There are so many things that they do not understand, it is difficult for them to explain and put their thoughts into any logical order.

The Bach Remedies are not going to miraculously patch their parents' marriage together again and make everything better, but they can certainly help the child cope with what is happening. One of the most important remedies is WALNUT because this remedy helps to protect against outside influences, and therefore protects the child from being drawn into the conflict. This remedy also assists periods of change and so it would help the child adjust to life with one parent instead of two. ASPEN is also a helpful remedy because of the dread of "something" about to happen; the sense of impending catastrophe. WHITE CHESTNUT is for persistent worrying thoughts, perhaps a re-occuring vision of losing a parent, and so is another very helpful remedy. In addition, AGRIMONY would help to ease the inner torment, agony, anxiety and fear that the child keeps hidden and does not want to talk about. Children who suffer like this often have disturbed restless nights – they may suffer with nightmares, crying out during sleep, sweating, tossing and turning, may talk during sleep or start to sleepwalk as their subconscious mind tries to release the pent up emotion. The stress has to go somewhere and if it cannot escape when the child is awake, then it will have another go when the child is asleep! Agrimony would help ease this hidden, unexpressed emotion, and ROCK ROSE would be useful if nightmares are a problem causing panic and terror. Some children cope with their fear by displaying bouts of problematic behaviour – aggression, pretending to be ill, telling lies, refusing to eat, being destructive, disobedient, rebellious or spiteful. It is, however, the *reason* for the behaviour – e.g. fear – that is the important consideration. Remedies such as VINE, HOLLY and CHICORY will help the behaviour, but remedies for the underlying fear are even more important.

Actual separation may be the worst part of all, or it may, in a way, be a relief because at least it means an end to the apprehension, the wondering and, most of all, the arguments, raised voices and unpleasantness. It is not surprising that children feel torn in two. They love both their parents, and are sometimes expected to take sides or make a choice between them. Some children begin to lose their confidence and identity and sense they are the object of argument. Then, like a tennis umpire, they silently watch the match go on, hearing one parent's argument and then the other, but whilst an umpire is fully aware and in tune with the state of play, the child presiding over *this* match is bewildered, uncertain and afraid. An end to this depressing situation may therefore come as a welcome relief; relaxation of the tension that has existed, and the hope that normality can be resumed to the home. Although many couples try to shield their children from the trauma by attempting to act "normally" in front of them, it is difficult to shield them completely, and children often sense there is something the matter, however hard you try to conceal it. Somehow, they just know.

The remedies are an invaluable support and those already mentioned may again be appropriate here, but there are others too which are perhaps particularly relevant when a separation actually takes place. WALNUT to help adjustment to the change in circumstances, SCLERANTHUS for the uncertainty, and CLEMATIS for the bewilderment. Some children blame themselves for the upset in the family. PINE would help children who blame themselves for the upset in the family or believe that if they had never been born, their parents would still be happy. ELM would help those who assume responsibility for what remains of the family and feel unable to cope with what is expected of them.

Whilst some children may be relieved when the conflict ends, despite parental separation, others will tolerate *anything* to keep their parents together. If separation is inevitable, much grief will understandably surround the disintegration of the family unit. The sadness, bewilderment and anger will naturally cause untold emotional agonies and the child may feel utterly helpless and empty. With regard to the remedies, STAR OF BETHLEHEM in particular would help to ease the shock and pain of grief, and soothe and comfort the sorrow. Naturally this would be extremely important for children whose parent has died, but would also help children who are coping with the loss of a parent from the home under any circumstance. Because thoughts of the past, haunting memories and recollections, can prevent the healing process from taking place, HONEYSUCKLE would be a helpful remedy too, and this would also help those who feel desperately homesick if they have had to move away. Some children bury their grief within themselves. They may hide behind a a protective barrier of enforced cheerfulness (AGRIMONY), or they may harbour a great deal of anger and become quarrelsome or defensive if the subject is raised, refusing to confront feelings and instead seek refuge behind a hostile exterior. It is natural to feel angry, and if this is expressed as hatred, a desperation to hit back at life, then HOLLY would help, or WILLOW to ease the bitterness – "why is life so unfair?", and resentment – "how could God be so unkind?"; VERVAIN would be helpful too for the sense of injustice, and WHITE CHESTNUT for the persistent mental arguments and sleeplessness; PINE if there should be any feelings of guilt or self-blame; SWEET CHESTNUT for the emptiness and despair as though nothing is worth living for any longer.

Sometimes children's emotions are directed at the remaining parent who will, in turn, be attempting to deal with his or her own grief. It is therefore important, no matter how hard it might be, for each member of the family to be strong in order to support one another.

HELP FOR THE PARENTS

So far, we have mainly concentrated on the effect of parental separation upon the child, but parents' own needs must not be forgotten. The remedies are for the whole family and there are several that can help. Much depends on individual character and temperament, but for the friction and tension that surrounds fraught situations perhaps the following would be useful: ELM for the feeling of being unable to cope. We usually associate Elm with being overwhelmed by responsibility at work, but the state of mind applies equally to responsibility at home – just the responsibility of life itself can be overwhelming at times. It is therefore an extremely important remedy when you lose sight of who is in control – when everything gets on top of you and you begin to feel you cannot cope with it anymore; BEECH for intolerance of one another; HOLLY for hatred, revenge, suspicion, jealousy – anger resulting from any of these emotions, perhaps connected with the "other man/woman", and for the spiteful temper that might follow; OLIVE for exhaustion or fatigue. This can be responsible for so many negative moods, because when we are over-tired, it may only take the smallest thing to tip the balance; PINE for the feelings of guilt which may occur – about the rift between you, about causing an upheaval for your children, blaming yourself for everything that has gone wrong. Similarly CRAB APPLE would help those who despise and condemn themselves for being wicked – cannot bear to look at themselves in the mirror because they see something evil in the reflection. This feeling is closely linked to Pine because it is frequently the guilt that causes the self-hatred. HONEYSUCKLE would help if there are regrets and a longing to turn back the clocks, wishing things could be as they once were; WALNUT would help you adjust to a new way of life; ROCK WATER and/or VINE for those who are in a situation which remains unresolved because neither party will back down! These remedies would help those who stubbornly refuse to give in – almost *forcing* themselves to be unhappy; VERVAIN would help those who will not give in because they are furious with the injustice of the whole situation – how *dare* he/she?; WHITE CHESTNUT for the mental arguments that inevitably take place.

There may also be a lot of doubt, lack of courage and uncertainty as to the course of action to take. WILD OAT will help those who feel they have reached a cross-roads in life and are not sure about their direction. MIMULUS will give courage to those who are afraid to follow the path of their own true convictions; LARCH for those who need more confidence in their ability to be successful on their own; CERATO for those who do not trust their intuition and so seek reassurance from others to confirm they are doing the right thing. SCLERANTHUS is for those who really do not know and come to a standstill because they cannot decide what to do for the best. For those who feel totally trapped and filled with despair, unable to see a reasonable way out, SWEET CHESTNUT is the remedy to soothe the heart and help some light to re-appear at the end of the tunnel, and STAR OF BETHLEHEM for the sadness felt by those who really do not want to separate, but do so because it seems the only solution.

IV	REJECTION

When we think about it, we all experience rejection of a sort at some time during our life. A broken relationship, failing a job interview or being turned down when inviting someone out, all result in a sense of rejection. Children may feel rejected by their peers at school – perhaps excluded from a certain group of friends, or ostracised for some reason. These feelings are quite common to most people, but the more fundamental rejection as a human being is naturally the most difficult to cope with.

Some children are rejected by their parents because the parents do not want them – maybe they never wanted to have children and have blamed the children rather than themselves for their birth. If parents are indifferent to the child and actively demonstrate those feelings, then the child is bound to develop a host of negative attitudes about himself – worthlessness, self-dislike, insecurity for example – and these may take such a strong-hold that they become ingrained on the child's character and are therefore difficult to eradicate later in life.

Sometimes, however, and maybe more usually, rejection is much more subtle, and may be characterised by constant criticism, verbal abuse and withheld approval or affection. Perhaps the parents have excessive expectations of the child who inevitably fails to measure up to their standards. This then results in low self esteem, guilt and under-valuation. The child himself may then react by becoming hostile and aggressive, or may develop a passive aggression, adopting a negative view of the world as a whole and withdraws into himself. The Bach Remedies can be of great help in any of these situations: PINE for feelings of guilt; CRAB APPLE for self condemnation or sense of worthlessness; LARCH for the low self-esteem and lack of self-confidence; CERATO for lack of self-belief, vulnerability and the desperate need for reassurance of the value of his personal existence. Indeed, many children do not believe they should even be alive. Again this feeling indicates guilt and so Pine *and* Cerato would help in combination. Conversely, WILLOW would help the child who blames others rather than himself – the child who resents his parents for what they have done, bears a grudge that cannot be shaken off, and may grow up with a big "chip on his shoulder", never being able to really forgive or forget. HOLLY is for the child who hates his parents.

Sometimes children who have had extremely strict parents who may have ruled their lives by instilling fear and wrath into their little minds, also grow up to be hard task-masters, rigid minded, self-denying and ruthless with themselves because they have grown up to believe that this is the *right* way to live. Such children would benefit from ROCK WATER which would help them to be kinder to themselves, to relax and allow themselves some pleasure in life, to know and realise that life is not intended to be sacrificial purgatory. Fear is often associated with this outlook and so remedies to deal with this would be helpful in addition.

Fear however is likely to be a problem in itself, especially if there has been disharmony within the home and there is a threat of broken relationships. What is going to happen to me? Where am I going to live? Am I going to be put into a home? Am I going to be punished? The main remedy for fear is MIMULUS as it is for all *known* fears. However, there may be a much greater fear, when the child is actually *terrified,* in which case ROCK ROSE would be a more appropriate remedy, or may be given in addition to Mimulus if necessary. Another remedy which is often required is ASPEN for anxiousness and apprehension for no specific reason – just a feeling of fear and trepidation that does not allow the child to really feel relaxed or safe. Some children may be afraid *for* their parents – what will happen to *them*? – RED CHESTNUT would be helpful for those who worry and fret over their parents' fate. Quite often these children are gentle, timid, easily dominated and will always do as they are told. It is their natural instinct to care, even under the most appalling circumstances. CENTAURY is the remedy to help children of this type find a greater inner strength. WALNUT would also be indicated in many cases because it is the remedy for protection against strong outside influences, and being the subject of any kind of disharmony or the victim of other people's negativity, Walnut would help to establish a protective barrier so that the child can remain true to himself.

V | **ADOPTION** We have already discussed how adoptive parents bond to their children and have just as much love to give and share as natural parents. But what about the children themselves? In their early years, if adopted as a baby, they will fit into family life and consider mum and dad as natural parents. It is when the child gets older and is told that he or she is adopted that doubts and queries may begin. Different children are bound to react in different ways. Some may not be interested in the past, concerned only with the family they know and love, whilst others will raise endless questions about who they really are. It is only natural for an adopted child to wonder who his or her real parents might be, what they look like, why they apparently "gave" their baby away, why they were "not wanted", and so on. It can affect the adoptive parents quite considerably, because all of a sudden, they may feel they have been pushed aside, and the natural parents whom the child does not even know, assume prime importance in the child's mind. It is not, however, because the child does not appreciate his adoptive parents, or does not want them any longer, but rather that he feels as though he is not the person he thought he was, as though he has led a life of pretence. He may even begin to question whether he deserves to exist at all. Sometimes adopted children begin to feel guilty, believe that they must have been horrible babies, for otherwise, they would not have been rejected. Sometimes they may feel very angry at everyone concerned, and frustrated because they do not know themselves any more, feel they have no family background or origins. We all tend to take our frustrations out on those whom we love the most, and so adoptive parents may similarly be the ones who have to bear the brunt of their child's emotional reaction. There are several remedies that can help children cope with their feelings:

STAR OF BETHLEHEM for the shock and subsequent grief for the life and family they do not know;
HOLLY for feelings of suspicion towards natural as well as adoptive parents. "I hate you for not telling me";
CERATO for questioning their right to be here, to life and existence – desperate for reassurance;
WILD OAT for the sense of being lost, of floundering, not knowing which way to turn, where to go, what life is all about…;
WHITE CHESTNUT for the mental arguments and persistent worrying thoughts.
PINE for feelings of guilt and self-blame;
WILLOW for feelings of resentment towards the natural parents for having abandoned them;

MIMULUS for feelings of fear that it is going to happen again, worried that the adoptive parents will abandon them as well.

Without a doubt, the whole situation needs to be dealt with tactfully with a great deal of patience and reassurance. Not all families will have problems – many will be able to accept it and adjust to it without difficulty, but for those whose children do feel upset, an understanding all round is vital to help them find the answers to their questions (they will not rest until they do!) in order to piece their life back together again and make sense of it. They will need to go through this process before being able to comfortably move forward and come to terms with the events of their life. With your help, they *will* achieve it and appreciate the warmth and quality of life you have together.

VI | OVER-PROTECTION

It is only natural for parents to want to protect their children – and indeed that is a vital parental role – but sometimes, perhaps due to over-concern for their welfare, parents or guardians may become *over*-protective and as a result, the child does not have the full opportunity to develop his own character or acquire complete autonomy because everything is done for him. It is usually quite unintentional on the part of the parents – it is only because they love their children that they want to do all they can for them – but the temptation is to do *too* much.

When the child grows up and reaches the age when he or she wants freedom and needs to be independent, if he has not learned how to do things for himself then it will be difficult for him to adapt. It may be that the growing child or teenager learns to actually *expect* things to be done for him, because that is what he has been used to. Boys, for example, who have never had to lift a finger in order to reap the benefits of eating a meal, wearing clean clothes, sleeping in a made bed or living in a clean home, frequently grow up to expect their wives to provide similar conditions – in effect, to "mother" them.

Over-protection is a trait that belongs to the remedy CHICORY which, at its most negative, turns love and the desire to help and be generous, into a selfish love which clings possessively to the family. The positive aspects of Chicory are positive indeed, and these type of people make the most loving and caring parents. Sometimes it is when they feel hurt because their children have turned against them or upset them in some way, that the balance to their nature is upset and the negative aspects begin to creep in. Maintaining equilibrium is the answer, and if you recognise yourself in the above, Chicory is the remedy to help you should you find yourself drifting into the habit of doing too much or "taking over".

It is difficult to believe that too much love can be a bad thing – it surely has to be better than too little – but children may feel stifled by it, as though they have to please their parents and conform to their wishes all the time, and as a result, do not get the opportunity to really get to know themselves, their skills, weaknesses and limitations, or what they truly want to gain from life. Before this happens, therefore, Chicory helps to redress the balance so that you can *all* live independently as individuals, enjoy each other's company and be able to receive love as well as give it. That way, a happy family relationship will flourish without any resentment or bitterness or danger of driving away those whom you care most about.

CHILD ABUSE

It is a sad fact of life that some children are subjected to cruelty, or are abused sexually. We seem to be constantly hearing about the plight of children who have been emotionally or physically injured and damaged, and in some cases killed, through neglect or violent attack. These cases are extreme, but nevertheless, child abuse, in whatever degree it takes place, does occur, and is something none of us can afford to ignore.

Physical abuse may mean anything from excessive smacking to bodily torture, and the accompanying emotional disturbances hardly need to be spelled out. Emotional deprivation too is a form of cruelty, and although there may be no obvious physical scars to show for it, it can be equally damaging.

There are two aspects to child abuse that we need to address – the cause and the effect. The reasons *why* children are abused is a question that, for most people, escapes comprehension, but no matter how we might feel towards those who have actively carried out such appalling cruelty, we cannot dismiss it out of hand. Some people are crying out for help and aiding them to overcome their emotional difficulties will be for everyone's good in the long run. For some people, it may be something that happens as a "one-off", and although this is no excuse, it may be due to a string of problems, traumas and difficulties that have got on top of the person concerned who has, in the end, "snapped" and taken it all out on the child. A mother who is finding it difficult to cope with three children under school-age and a young baby who never stops screaming, may reach a certain pitch that she cannot take it any longer, and the next time the baby cries she is overcome with an urge to smother it, violently shake it or lash out at it. She may well regret it afterwards, but this is no help to the injured child. What is important in circumstances like this is the *prevention* of the situation in the first place, and whilst she may need professional psychological help and support as well as that of her partner and family, the remedies have a role to play too. ELM, for example, would help her not to lose sight of her ability to cope. CHERRY PLUM would help the loss of control; the sudden compelling urge to injure her child, HOLLY the spite and hate-filled anger.

There are some people, however, who simply have a sadistic streak, and therefore enjoy inflicting pain, even on an innocent child. Unfortunately these people rarely come forward for help, at least not until some time after the event when perhaps they realise what they have done and are filled with remorse. There is not therefore always the opportunity to resolve a situation, or at the very least, take the heat out of it, and thus avoid the escalation to violence.

Sexual abuse of children is something that has made the news headlines on several occasions, especially in more recent years. One hears of stories where a father has sexually abused his daughter(s), or even his son(s), but equally, the abuser may be an older brother, uncle, baby-sitter, child-minder or female relative. Sometimes sexual abuse can take a physically violent form, but often it is something that starts more subtly at a young age, the abuser winning the co-operation of the child by telling him or her that it is a game. There may come a point, however, when the child knows that what is going on is not right, becomes afraid and begins to protest, but is subjected to threats of punishment if he or she tells anyone. The child is then left to worry and fret, feeling terrified of what is going on, terrified of the punishing threats and yet desperate to make it stop. When a child *does* speak out, the abuser will emphatically deny it and the child then not only has to continue to be abused, but punished as well and regarded as a liar. Sadly, some children are subjected to these horrific ordeals time and time again, month after month, year after year, until eventually someone takes notice of them.

Unfortunately the emotional scars of sexual abuse can be long lasting, causing insurmountable difficulties when the child grows up and reaches the age when boy/girl relationships take place. The emotional consequences may indeed last a lifetime. The remedies therefore, given as soon as possible, would help to ease the pain, at least a little, so that the child stands a chance of establishing some form of normal rhythm to his or her life.

TERROR – the remedy to help this is ROCK ROSE. It is also an ingredient of the Rescue Remedy which may be given as an alternative. Terror is one of the most profound emotions experienced by those subjected to abuse of any nature, and may create terrifying thoughts about men, the abuser, punishment, subsequent consequences, and also may be the cause of nightmares.

SHOCK – this too is naturally going to be apparent. Shock to the system of the abuse – the first time it happens as well as the whole on-going affair. The remedy for shock is STAR OF BETHLEHEM. This too is contained in the Rescue Remedy and because shock and terror are so often linked, **Rescue Remedy** may be more suitable to alleviate the initial impact of the traumatic ordeal.

GUILT – very often, children blame themselves and feel guilty about what has happened. If they should feel this way, PINE is the remedy to help them to appreciate that it is not their fault.

DISGUST – a sense of self-disgust is often accompanied by guilt, but feeling dirty, contaminated, interfered with or violated, can be horrendously distressing and may lead to despair or obsessive behaviour. CRAB APPLE is the remedy that will help any child who feels disgusted in this way.

FEAR – in addition to the terror and panic that would be evident, there is also likely to be an underlying fear and nervousness. A constant sense of apprehension about what might happen, worrying about if and when it will happen again. MIMULUS is the remedy to help known fears, and ASPEN for unknown fears, anxiousness and a feeling of uneasiness. Both remedies may be required together.

DOMINATION – understandably, children who are subjected to cruelty or sexual abuse are going to feel threatened and dominated. Together with the fear they are experiencing, they may also be unable to stand up to the control of the abuser and so find themselves having to give in to his (or her) demands time after time. CENTAURY is the remedy for children of a kind, gentle, easily dominated nature, but would help any child who felt they were being manipulated and controlled and unable to withstand it.

DESPAIR – any of these emotions may well lead to a sense of despair, a feeling as though there is no way out of the misery. The remedy for this anguish is SWEET CHESTNUT.

UNCERTAINTY – the child may express doubt about what to do, whether or not he should report the abuser. If he is hesitant, SCLERANTHUS would help him to make the right decision.

WORRY – anything that is distressing creates worrying thoughts, mental arguments and constant mental stress. These thoughts may keep sufferers awake at night, or they may be able to forget them and so sleep soundly, only to be reminded once again when they wake up. WHITE CHESTNUT is the remedy to help ease the incessant mental torment that worry can cause.

HIDDEN EMOTIONS – because of the nature of the situation, many children keep it all to themselves. They do not tell a soul and so suffer inner agonies that are, understandably, extremely difficult for them to bear. If they are able to remain strong and brave and not let it get the better of them, then they would be OAK children, but usually the exterior appearance of "normality" is a façade – a front that they have established because they do not want to make a fuss and so try not to let anyone see how they are suffering. AGRIMONY is the remedy to help these children. Unfortunately, because they are able to conceal their emotions so well, their pain often goes unnoticed. However, sometimes one may see a glimpse of emotion despite the carefree attitude, or intuitively sense their anguish. The remedy can then be given to ease the inner torment and help them to be able to release it and share it so that they will, hopefully, receive the help they so desperately need.

❧ ❧

Emotional deprivation is a form of child abuse that often escapes recognition. There are no bruises or marks on the skin and so it frequently goes unnoticed. Nevertheless, neglect of a child's emotional needs can have just as much impact on their health and well-being as physical neglect. Love may be difficult to explain, but it is an essential ingredient of happiness, and so if children are deprived of parental love or the substitute love of their guardian, then they will grow up to feel hollow and find it difficult to cope with giving and/or receiving it in future relationships. We have already discussed how a child may feel rejected when his or her parents are facing marital difficulties, and similar emotions are generated in the situation in which a child is subjected to emotional deprivation. Similar remedies therefore will be required in this case, particularly STAR OF BETHLEHEM for the sense of loss or grief, CERATO for the search for reassurance, and CHICORY for the desperate need to love and be loved.

It is, however, as with any other situation, essential to treat the child as an individual. I have offered some remedy suggestions, but because every child is different, each one must be considered separately and remedies chosen according to their specific needs. The remedies, because they offer comfort and support to help children gain the mental strength to cope with their difficulties, are therefore of immense value to children who have been subjected to the anguish associated with physical pain and suffering, those who have been deprived of love and affection, and those who have suffered the horror of sexual abuse.

CHAPTER 5

Health and Illness

CHILDHOOD IS A PERIOD when one infectious disease can be expected after another. Whilst the Bach Remedies are not a treatment for disease as such, by helping children feel stronger emotionally, they will feel better in themselves, and this will encourage their whole system to recover more quickly.

I | **WHEN CHILDREN ARE ILL**

A baby is born with some passively inherited immunity from its mother, and babies who are breast fed receive certain antibodies through breast milk. These antibodies help to protect them during their first weeks of life and help to build a resistance to allergic conditions such as asthma and eczema. It does not, however, last forever.

There are numerous strains of viruses that can cause ill health, so babies and children become ill from time to time, and even though you may feel the problem is trivial, if you are at all concerned, it is always best to seek advice from one of the primary health care team, your child care clinic or family doctor who will either offer appropriate treatment or reassure you that all is well. Either way, it is without a doubt, better to be safe than sorry!

The Bach Remedies are not a treatment for physical conditions or for diseases as such, and they are not a substitute for necessary medical treatment. Clearly, if a child has a raging infection then some specific medicine is required to deal with it, whether it be from an orthodox or homoeopathic doctor. The Bach Remedies however, can assist the healing process by easing the associated emotional traumas and encouraging a return of equilibrium. Whatever the illness, as far as your choice of Bach Remedies is concerned, the basis for selection lies in the emotional outlook and mood of the child. Dr. Bach gave a perfect example of this during a lecture given on his birthday, September 24th 1936, two months before he died. He said:

"We all know the same illness may take us quite differently: if Tommy gets measles, he may be irritable, Sissy may be quiet and drowsy, Johnny wants to be petted, little Peter may be all nerves and fearful, Bobbie wants to be left alone, and so on.

Now if disease has such different effects, it is certain it is no use treating the disease alone; it is better to treat Tommy, Sissy, Johnny, Peter and Bobbie and get them each well, and then "good-bye" the measles.

What is important to impress upon you is that it is not the measles which gives the guide to the cure, but it is the way the little one is affected: and the mood of the little one is the most sensitive guide as to know what that particular patient needs.

And just as moods guide us to the treatment in illness, so also they may warn us ahead of a complaint approaching and enable us to stop the attack.

Little Tommy comes home from school unusually tired, or drowsy or irritable, or wanting to be fussed, or perhaps left alone and so on. He is "not quite himself" as we say. Kind neighbours come in and say "Tommy is sickening for something, you will have to wait". But why wait: if Tommy is treated then according to his mood, he may very soon again be turned from "not quite himself" into "quite himself", when whatever illness was threatened will not occur.

And so with any of us: before almost all complaints there is usually a time of not being quite fit or a bit run down: that is the time to treat our condition, get fit and stop things going any further.

Prevention is better than cure, and these remedies help us in a wonderful way to get well, and to protect ourselves from attack of things unpleasant."

There are, nevertheless, certain remedies that can help in specific ways, and occasions when we can apply some of the remedies to relieve certain symptoms. The irritation of the skin caused by chicken pox for example, can be greatly soothed by the application of the **Rescue Remedy Cream.** A lotion may also be applied to any external irritation or soreness – a few drops of **Rescue Remedy** and **Crab Apple,** for its cleansing properties, in a little lukewarm boiled water, and then applied with cotton wool to the skin, also has very soothing and healing advantages. A compress of a similar lotion may also be applied to the forehead, chest, neck and wrists, and remedies specific to the child's personal needs (as well as Rescue Remedy if necessary) may be given in a drink to help re-establish a calm frame of mind and so enhance recovery.

Illness is draining – it depletes our energy – and OLIVE being the remedy for exhaustion, helps the system to regain that lost energy and find the strength to fight disease and get well. If we consider Dr. Bach's example of Tommy, Sissy, Johnny, Peter and Bobbie, the remedies that would be appropriate for them would be IMPATIENS for Tommy (irritable), CLEMATIS for Sissy (quiet and drowsy), CHICORY for Johnny (wants to be petted), MIMULUS for Peter (all nerves and fearful), and WATER VIOLET for Bobbie (wants to be left alone). All these children are suffering from the same disease, in this case measles, and yet would, in Bach Remedy terms, all require different remedies.

WILLOW is a remedy that is also often called upon in times of illness. It is for those who feel sorry for themselves and is also for those who resent being ill. It is very natural, for example, if you are in pain and suitable sympathy is not forthcoming, to begin to feel resentful and self-pitying, but if we can recognise it in ourselves, or in our children, then the Willow remedy is there to help to lift that depressing inward negativity so that a much more positive outlook is formed. This in itself will help to take one's mind off the pain or feeling of malaise so that it no longer seems quite so severe, to be able to cope with it more easily, and to be positive and hopeful about being well again. CHICORY would help children who "cling" or become "whiny" when ill and want to be constantly attended to. It may be that Chicory and Willow are needed together. A child who seems to be revelling in his illness, not really wanting to be well, maybe pretending he is still ill long after he is better, because he enjoys the attention it brings him and all the fuss that is made, would also indicate CHICORY, but HEATHER would be useful for hypochondria and the enjoyment of being ill. Heather children are likely to describe how they feel in graphic detail, over and over again, providing a full account to anyone who will listen.

Children generally, however, will not continue to be "ill" longer than they have to. As soon as they are feeling well in themselves, even though their body may still be covered in spots, they will want to be out of bed and playing, resuming normality. Children's illnesses do not, usually, linger as long as they would during adulthood, partly because of their youth and ability to recover more speedily, but also because their state of mind is more open and carefree.

| COMMON AILMENTS | Coughs and colds are common to us all and I doubt if there are

many people who have managed to escape a cold altogether. Although they are common and are usually relatively minor illnesses, colds are nevertheless, uncomfortable and can be utterly miserable, especially for a child. Being blocked up with mucus, finding it hard to breath properly, feeling tired and thick-headed is enough to make even the most placid child irritable, and although the Bach Remedies do not actually treat the cold itself, they can certainly help the accompanying moods.

CRAB APPLE is a helpful remedy in all cases of illness because it is for cleansing, and will therefore help to eradicate the "diseased feeling". Other remedies that are helpful depend on the individual child's mood and temperament, but some common remedies when a child is poorly with a cold are: HORNBEAM for the lack of energy, feeling of weariness and lethargy, cannot be bothered to get up or have a wash or eat anything; WILD ROSE for the apathy that causes some children to simply resign themselves to being ill and lose interest in actively trying to get better. OLIVE, as already described, is the remedy for *actual* tiredness, and any illness will deplete the body of energy, so Olive would be supportive in a return to health by helping the child regain his or her strength. Because colds so often cause sufferers to feel miserable, sorry for themselves and seek sympathy, WILLOW, CHICORY and HEATHER as described previously would also be useful remedies to consider.

Some children may be frightened, especially if a blocked nose makes it difficult to breath, particularly at night. RESCUE REMEDY is probably the best remedy if the child becomes panicky, but MIMULUS would be appropriate for more general fears. Mimulus is the remedy for shy or nervous children who are, by nature, afraid of all sorts of things. In illness, these children become afraid of being ill, afraid they will suffocate, afraid of vomiting and so on.

Children who become bad tempered and cross when ill would be helped with IMPATIENS for irritability, and BEECH for annoyance and intolerance.

It may also be helpful to put some of the remedies into the child's bath water – **Olive, Crab Apple and Rescue Remedy** particularly (about 10 drops of each), and if the child has a temperature, a lotion of a few drops of the appropriate remedies diluted in cool water and applied to the forehead with a flannel as a compress, will be soothing too.

Very young babies are "nose breathers", and so colds can be quite serious if their nose becomes blocked and so it would always be advisable to see your doctor if your baby has a cold, as some other treatment or advice may be more appropriate for your particular infant. A baby who is finding it hard to breath through a stuffed up nose is likely to be restless and irritable, frustrated by the symptoms it does not understand. This may be most noticeable during feed times because although babies have an uncanny knack of being able to breathe, feed and vocalise simultaneously, if they can't breathe then they are not going to be able to feed comfortably either. RESCUE REMEDY would be the most appropriate remedy for the relief of the agitated state of mind.

III | **ALLERGIES** | Very often children with allergic reactions, whether it be asthma, hay fever or eczema, feel worse when something is troubling them – prior to an examination, or if they are having problems with school-work, a teacher or another pupil, or there is a stressful situation at home.

We all have personal weaknesses, and when we are worried about something, tired, upset, depressed or generally not feeling "ourselves", then whatever our "weakness" might be; skin problems, migraine, asthma attacks, digestive disturbances, or hay fever, it tends to worsen. In a way, these constitutional weaknesses are the body's natural release because when there has been a build up of stress, something has to eventually give way. Some people are better at releasing it than others and some people never seem to suffer physically at all, whereas others seem to be prone to some form of physical difficulty all their lives.

Allergies such as hay fever, eczema and asthma are associated with a variety of substances and suggested causes. House dust, cat hair, certain foodstuffs, for example, are related to and regarded as being responsible for asthma attacks. We should, however, consider why it is that some children suffer with asthma when exposed to cats or house dust, whilst others do not, and why some children suffer with terrible hay fever when exposed to pollen whilst others can play happily in long grass and not even sneeze. The true *cause* of the allergy, must lie in the make-up of the individual child. It is therefore important to be aware of the personality, moods and emotional outlook of each one in order to select remedies accurately. In Bach Remedy terms, we need to find the "type remedy". We cannot generalise and offer a combination to suit all needs. Each child must be assessed separately so that his or her own personal remedies can be identified.

HAY FEVER

Hay fever can be a most distressing and uncomfortable complaint which makes summer time absolute misery. Some people do not suffer until they reach adulthood, but it is more common to develop hay fever in childhood and then "grow out" of it, and although it may always remain a weakness to a certain extent, symptoms generally tend to decrease as life goes on.

Classic hay fever symptoms include sneezing, a tickling throat, a blocked yet streaming nose, itchy swollen eyes, fatigue, wheeziness (which may cause an acute attack of asthma), and coughing. RESCUE REMEDY is always beneficial to have for the urgency of the situation, but CRAB APPLE is also recommended, being the cleansing remedy. Crab Apple and Rescue Remedy can be taken orally as well as applied, diluted, externally to the eyes (either on eye-pads soaked in a dilution of the remedies and water, or in an eye bath). This can help to ease the irritating symptoms and thus help to soothe the sore and puffy eyes. OLIVE is another very helpful remedy – it is for tiredness and fatigue, and again may be added to an external application if desired as well as given orally. If the child is old enough, a gargle containing Rescue Remedy and Crab Apple would also be helpful if an irritating throat is a nuisance.

❀ ECZEMA

This irritating and sometimes painful skin complaint can begin in babyhood. Quite often it is relatively short lasting, the child growing out of it before reaching school age. Others however, suffer throughout childhood and sometimes during adulthood as well. It usually appears in the elbow and knee creases, around the neck and in the groin. Some children suffer with it extensively, covering their face, neck and hands, and when it is visible it is infinitely more uncomfortable and distressing than when it is hidden because the sufferer is often embarrassed about the complaint. This can be compounded by the tactlessness of people who may cringe away from close contact with an eczema sufferer. Whispers, jeers and sneering remarks can be desperately hard to cope with, and because eczema, as with other allergic conditions, is frequently stress related, may in turn exacerbate the problem because ridicule itself is stressful – as if the eczema alone wasn't bad enough! Bach Remedies directed at the way the child feels, therefore, will help to break into this cycle so that he or she is less upset, agitated or depressed.

There are, however, other factors which may also be to blame – fabric conditions, soap-powders, certain clothing materials, or shampoo for example – so it is always good practice to eliminate these potential culprits first, rather than assume the eczema is caused by stress alone. If the child *is* emotionally upset by something, however, the Bach Remedies can help enormously by gently easing the stress so that the child's system can begin its own healing. RESCUE REMEDY is a good all-round calming remedy, but CRAB APPLE is also important as it comforts the minds of children who are troubled or obsessed with what they look like; *feeling* diseased or ugly. GENTIAN would help those children who become depressed about the complaint, or by the attitude of other children, and WALNUT to help protect them from these influences. CENTAURY will help the child who is easily dominated and thus lacks the strength to stand up to others; CERATO for the child who needs to be reassured and doubts him or herself; LARCH for the child who lacks confidence; MIMULUS for the child who is fearful, and

WILLOW for the child who withdraws into himself, feels sorry for himself or resents other people who do not suffer the way he does.

VERVAIN children are highly strung, tense, unrelaxed, and always on the go. IMPATIENS children are short tempered, quick off the mark, always hurrying, impatient with slowness. This remedy also helps the irritation in the mind caused by the irritating skin. AGRIMONY is for the child who pretends nothing troubles him, but hides his anguish behind a cheery façade. It would not be obvious to most people that anything is wrong, and even though the parents may sense that something is the matter, cannot quite ascertain what it is, and so Agrimony children by virtue of the way they are, may suffer considerable inner agonies. WATER VIOLET children also hide their feelings, but not in the same way as an Agrimony child. Water Violets tend to simply keep themselves to themselves and become aloof in response to other children's attitudes, adopting a superiority to protect them from hurtful remarks. ROCK WATER children would be self-sacrificing in their attempts to rid their system of the "disease".

An external application of certain remedies may also help relieve the irritation and soreness. RESCUE REMEDY CREAM would be an ideal choice as it is both soothing and generally healing. There are, however, some eczemas that do not respond well to *any* cream, so a lotion made up from drops of the remedy diluted in lukewarm water and dabbed onto the affected areas with cotton wool may be preferable. Rescue Remedy would again be helpful, together with Crab Apple – these two offering an ideal composite. There have been numerous good reports from adult sufferers as well as from parents who have found the remedies applied externally in this way successful for their children. Rescue Remedy Cream is usually what the good results of topical use are attributed to, and generally it has proved to be extremely helpful.

❧ ASTHMA

One of the most common conditions of childhood is asthma. Some-times asthmatic children will suffer with the condition throughout their adult lives as well, but usually it becomes less severe as they get older. Asthma means "wheezing" – the expiratory noise caused by spasm of the muscle wall which narrows the bronchial passages. The wheezing is worse during expiration and leaves the sufferer gasping for breath.

We have to breathe because our life depends on oxygen. This is rather an obvious statement, but one that is absolutely crucial to understanding asthma. Our body takes the oxygen and produces in return, its waste gas, carbon dioxide. The build up of carbon dioxide in the blood stream sends a signal to the brain which in turn triggers the expansion of the lungs, and as the lungs expand, air is drawn in through the nose or mouth. Because asthmatics have difficulty breathing *out*, they have an increasing amount of carbon dioxide building up in their system which acts as stimulation to breathe *in* again. The result being that their lungs go into spasm, and the constriction of the air passages makes it difficult for them to breathe at all. They are gasping because of their need for oxygen, but cannot rid their system of excess carbon dioxide. They therefore start to suffocate on their own inhalations, a very frightening thing to experience.

RESCUE REMEDY, because its five ingredients help to ease terror and panic, loss of control, hysteria, shock, irritation and agitation, may help to dilute the crisis by bringing about a more relaxed frame of mind. It should be emphasised, however, that Rescue Remedy is not a specific treatment for asthma, and although it is an excellent supportive measure, does not replace medication or emergency treatment.

A bout of asthma attacks is frequently attributed to stressful circumstances, and so in addition to treating the child constitutionally with his or her personal type remedy, it is also important to help the moods related to the cause of the stress. For example, a particular sufferer may be a shy nervous type of child – that would indicate MIMULUS – but an attack is provoked because the child moved house and had to settle into a new school. This would require WALNUT, the remedy for change and adjustment. In addition to this, the child may be experiencing restless nights because he/she is worrying about making new friends, finding his way round an unfamiliar building and whether or not the teachers will be friendly. For these worrying thoughts WHITE CHESTNUT would be indicated to calm the troubled mind. A combination of all three remedies would therefore be appropriate for this particular child in this particular situation. Another child who is also starting a new school, may be quite different – he may appear to be confident, even arrogant, yet underneath may be hiding his true feelings and trembling inside. This child may be sleeping soundly but restless nevertheless, perhaps waking momentarily with nightmarish dreams. This child would also require WALNUT for the change in circumstances, but would not necessarily require Mimulus or White Chestnut. The situation described here would be more indicative of AGRIMONY because this child is putting on a brave confident face and so this remedy would help to relieve the inner torture, and ROCK ROSE for the distress of nightmares.

V | SERIOUS ILLNESS

Children often seem to cope with a distressing diagnosis or prognosis remarkably well. This may be because they do not have the same sense of danger that adults might have. Generally, children are much braver. They will happily climb trees, for example, without any fear of falling, and are indeed excited by "dangerous" acts such as walking on a high wall, rolling down a steep hill, or swinging precariously upside down from a climbing frame – these things never seem to worry them. Activities that would make adults feel quite giddy, children tend to find thrilling! When they are ill, therefore, a similar fearlessness is often apparent and it is because of this that they are perhaps able to approach it, accept it and cope with it in a philosophical manner, often to the surprise of family and friends who are having difficulty coping with their own feelings.

Nevertheless, there are bound to be moments when fear, anxiety and sadness will fill their thoughts. The remedies can gently help them to deal with these emotions so that a positive state of mind has a chance to return. The individuality of the child is very important in choosing the right remedies, because it is the child's personality that is the "balancing factor", but here is a selection of some that are perhaps the most commonly called upon, specifically in relation to sick children:

FEAR AND ANXIOUSNESS – MIMULUS would help those who are nervous and afraid. They may be afraid of investigations, procedures, hospitals, doctors, pain and being sick. Mimulus is the remedy to help ease any known fear of this nature. It is also the personal remedy for children who are shy and timid, afraid of strangers and strange places, and may feel frightened if left unattended, or afraid to leave their parents.

ASPEN would help the child who feels uneasy, suffering with an unexplained apprehension; fearful, but not really knowing why.

AGRIMONY would help the child who keeps smiling and seems to cope, but underneath, does not feel as strong as he might appear. Agrimony will help relieve the inner pain and anxiety that he harbours.

CHERRY PLUM would help the child who suffers with sudden moments of panic, hysteria etc. It may be combined with ROCK ROSE which is the remedy for terror, or given as Rescue Remedy. Its action will be to bring calm to the troubled mind.

GUILT – PINE is for the child who feels guilty and blames himself for being ill, for putting everyone to so much trouble and so on. The Pine child apologises if he is sick, apologises for making the bed dirty or untidy, is always saying "I'm sorry" even for things that are beyond his control or not his fault at all.

SHOCK AND GRIEF – STAR OF BETHLEHEM is for the child who has received a shock – this may be in the form of serious news, or it may be the shock to the system of an operation, uncomfortable medical procedures or particular treatment. Star of Bethlehem is also the remedy for grief and sorrow, and a child who knows that he is seriously ill, or even terminally ill, may begin to grieve for his family, for life and feel a harrowing sense of sadness. Star of Bethlehem is the remedy to comfort him in his distress, and help him to heal the wound in his heart.

ADJUSTMENT – WALNUT is for the child who is finding it difficult to come to terms with his illness. It may be something that is going to alter his quality of life having to rely on crutches or a wheelchair for example – and he is finding it difficult to adjust to the idea of having to live differently. Walnut is the remedy for changes in circumstances and is a link-breaker so helps the child to make the step forward to get on positively with the life that lies ahead of him.

Walnut would also help to ease any transitional adjustment and help the child come to terms with the prognosis of his particular illness.

CRAB APPLE would help the child who feels that his body is diseased, feels contaminated by the ailment and becomes obsessed with it. Crab Apple would help to relieve the mind of these thoughts.

STRENGTH OF CHARACTER – VINE is for the child who is very strong-willed; the child who tends to order people around, stubbornly refuses to do as he is told, will not allow nurses/doctors/parents to tend to him. This attitude can cause a lot of tension which only stands in the way of the child making a recovery, so the Vine remedy will help a child of this nature to relax and be more accepting of help, and allow others who, on this occasion, *do* know better, to be in charge of him for a change.

WATER VIOLET will help those who keep themselves to themselves, speak little of their problems or illness. They are private individuals who hide their feelings, not in a jovial way as an Agrimony would do, but in an honest and dignified way. Water Violet children want to be left alone when they are ill, do not want to have people fussing around them, hate being examined or tended to, and will try to cover themselves up if there is a threat of exposure. The Water Violet remedy would help children of this nature to relax the shield they put around themselves, so that they can let other people in, just for a while, to bring comfort and reassurance.

OAK would help the child who does not *pretend* to be brave as the Agrimony child would do, but who *is genuinely* brave, and therefore does not become depressed or down-hearted. Oak people keep going, no matter what adversity might come their way, and never give up or give in. The remedy would help a child of this nature, should he begin to lose that inner strength or feel frustrated, to regain the determination to continue to fight.

DISINTEREST AND WITHDRAWAL – GORSE is for the child who has lost his fighting spirit; the child who has given up hope. It will help to reverse the negative pessimism so that a more positive and optimistic outlook returns.

SWEET CHESTNUT is for the child who feels at his wits end as to what to do. He feels utterly desolate as though there is little to live for. Sweet Chestnut will help to soothe the heart and allow a glimmer of hope to appear once again.

WILD ROSE is for the child who has not so much given *up*, but given *in* to his illness, become resigned to it and becomes apathetic towards doing anything to make himself feel better. Wild Rose will help a child who feels this way to be more enthusiastic about life, and to help him find some motivation to do something positive to help himself.

WILLOW is for the child who feels sorry for himself, resents others, blames them for his ill-health. For the child who becomes sulky and sullen and withdraws into an introspectively negative self-pity. The remedy will help him to think about something other than his own unhappiness, to help him feel more optimistic about life generally, and to use his energy to fight the illness rather than fight those who are trying to help him.

CLEMATIS is for the child who loses interest in the present because his thoughts are "wandering". He is not "grounded" and tends to day-dream, sleeps a lot, lacks concentration, and thinks only of the future, a fantasy or drifts into a state of mental oblivion. Clematis helps children of this nature to concentrate on the present as well as what might be to follow, so that life *now* becomes important once more.

OLIVE would help the child who feels tired and exhausted. This is likely to be a remedy that will apply to most children who are ill, because illness itself is draining. Olive is the remedy to help the child overcome his fatigue during illness as well as in the recuperative period.

HORNBEAM would help the child who feels lethargic, heavy, has a lack of motivation to get up in the morning, get dressed or look ahead to the day in front of him. Hornbeam would help to give a child who feels like this more enthusiasm for living, and this will also help him to regain his fighting spirit.

| V | **COPING WITH A CHILD'S DEATH** |

It goes without saying that a serious or terminal illness is going to be far more distressing than one which causes only minor concern. Many serious and potentially life threatening illnesses are now thankfully either preventable by way of immunisation, or treatable. Medical research is constantly striving to find cures, and whilst it is successful in many cases some diseases seem to constantly evade a techno-scientific solution. Science does, however, look at disease in an earthbound, material way, and the objective seems to be to cure and maintain physical life at all costs. As a human being, survival and the desire to live and be healthy is natural, but if we consider the spiritual implications, disease of physical matter does not seem so important. Accepting life on a wider plane than this earthly existence alone, however, is difficult and requires faith in the existence of spirituality and belief in the Life Force that makes True Life eternal. Not everyone has that faith and so when faced with death of the human body, it is, to some, the end of life, and naturally much harder to come to terms with.

Sometimes children are born with a condition that means their life will be short, or they may become chronically or terminally ill during infancy. Parents may have a chance to prepare themselves, although it does not make the initial shock and subsequent worry any easier. Grief will be no less painful for the parent who has lost their child through chronic disease as for a parent who has experienced the trauma of losing a child after a fatal accident or acute illness. The grieving process is the same, and follows a similar pattern whatever the circumstances might be.

The Bach Remedies cannot change the circumstances or turn back the clocks, but they can help to ease the transition, at least a little, and offer a gentle helping hand to guide you through it. The following remedies may be appropriate to help you cope throughout the various grieving stages. STAR OF BETHLEHEM is the comforting remedy, so would help to ease the shock and intense sorrow. Fear is also very common – fear of not coping (MIMULUS); hysterical fears of never being able to recover (CHERRY PLUM); fear that another child in the family might die or become seriously ill (RED CHESTNUT); fear of the unknown, an uneasy sensation of apprehension and morbid foreboding (ASPEN), or absolute terror and panic about some future fate (ROCK ROSE).

Guilt is a very common and sometimes disastrous emotion because it has a corrosive habit of turning inward, eating away at any rational thought, protection or self esteem that you might have left, leaving you condemning yourself for something that really you had no control over. But thoughts like "why didn't I do so and so...", and "if only I had called the doctor sooner...", tend to prey on the mind and if they continue for long they will end up convincing you that you *were* wrong, that you *are* to blame and as you become more and more convinced, so the emotional quick-sand thickens and then you find yourself sinking deeper and deeper into it. The remedy to help pull you out, or better still, stop you slipping into it in the beginning, is PINE, the remedy for guilt. HONEYSUCKLE would also help ease distressing regrets of the past – "if only" and "I wish" – and encourage the mind to look forward. Guilt is sometimes expressed as anger. WILLOW would help to ease the feeling of resentment – blaming the hospital, doctor or health visitor for not having done something to save the child. Blaming one's partner for not having been at home often enough, or not helping around the house or giving the children sufficient time and attention. Some men may even blame their partners for not having breast fed. Willow, in all these cases, is the remedy to help one appreciate that no single person or situation or circumstance is to blame. It is a difficult thing to accept because somehow it helps to relieve one's own self-blame if it can be pinned to someone else. Sometimes, therefore, Pine will be needed as well as Willow.

If anger is due to hatred or a desire for revenge, then HOLLY would be indicated, or VERVAIN if you believe there was malpractice and feel you must formally complain, and are therefore angry due to the injustice.

During the period of deep grief, there is sometimes a tendency to withdraw and either break or lose social contacts. This is where WATER VIOLET would be helpful as it is for those who grieve silently and alone.

There are, however, bound to be occasions when depression descends, perhaps a feeling of despair about ever being happy again. SWEET CHESTNUT is for this feeling. It will warm the heart and gently relieve the agonising despair that so hurts the mind and tortures the thoughts.

Pangs of anger and sadness will be sparked off from time to time when something serves as a painful reminder, and the period of recovery can take a long time, maybe several years. You will never forget, and you will never want to forget, but the trauma will gradually become easier, and although it is a very well-worn cliché, time really is a good healer.

Children with
Extra Special Needs

CHILDREN WHO ARE BORN WITH or who acquire by illness or accident, a disability are often referred to as being "handicapped" or "disadvantaged", but what do these terms really mean? Anything that prevents a child from reaching developmental milestones or leading a fully able-bodied life may be considered to be a handicap, but how far do we take it? Are only *disabled* children handicapped? Are all handicapped children necessarily disadvantaged? A child with diabetes is restricted in certain ways, but is a diabetic child a handicapped child? It is a wide question and one for which we will probably never find a satisfactory answer. As far as the Bach Remedies are concerned, it really does not matter what the "handicap" or "disability" is because they do not treat the condition, but in order to relieve the emotional distress suffered by many children, the personality and emotional outlook are the guiding factors and will apply regardless of the condition. Let us, nevertheless, consider as examples, *some* of the difficulties, both physical and mental, that are disabling, and how the remedies can help not only the children concerned, but their families too.

I

THE NEEDS OF THE FAMILY

Raising a child with a disabling handicap can put any family under a great deal of pressure, and create certain problems in relation to normal family life. Going on holiday, for example, may need more careful thought than it would do otherwise; finding out whether the resort, hotel or accommodation has the necessary facilities, and so on. A mother who has planned to go back to work after her baby is born may have to change her plans, and the father may need to take time off work. The family may also suffer ostracism, perhaps because they live in an isolated community with no local support. These are just a few of the problems that a family with a handicapped member may have to face, but there are also plenty of routine day-to-day activities that are restricted or require a different approach and can make daily living an obstacle course.

Every parent responds differently to the responsibility that lies before them. When the baby is first born some may have agonised over what they should do for the best, whilst for others there would have been no question about it at all. There may have been a chance to come to terms with the idea of bringing up a handicapped child during pregnancy, or it may have been a complete shock. Whether there had been a confirmed diagnosis or only intuitive suspicion, it is probably true to say that one never stops hoping that the baby will be healthy after all. Either way, there is bound to be an element of shock at first and a natural period of grief for the loss of the normal child you had expected or at least hoped for. Shock, disbelief, anger and guilt are only some of the emotions that may be experienced, and so the Bach Remedies can really be a tower of strength during this difficult period.

STAR OF BETHLEHEM would help to ease the shock associated with the initial confrontation with the truth and the grief and sadness associated with the death of a dream. VERVAIN would help the sense of injustice, the fury over how unfair life is. These feelings often lead to anger and frustration causing relentless mental arguments and other thoughts going round and round in the mind. WHITE CHESTNUT would help to ease these persistent thoughts, and WILLOW would help the resentment and bitterness if the feeling is more inward – a festering grudge against life, God and mothers who are happily nursing perfectly normal babies. HOLLY would help to ease any jealousy that you might have towards other mothers and families, and it would also ease feelings of hatred which may be directed towards the midwife who delivered your baby, the doctors, your partner, or even your new-born child. PINE helps to ease the feelings of guilt which may be related to thoughts such as "can I love this child as much as I should?" or "can I love this child as much as my other children?". Sometimes there is a strong feeling of protection, intermixed with a feeling of revulsion. The revulsion would be helped with CRAB APPLE as it is the cleansing remedy and will help you to get thoughts that make you shudder out of your mind. The guilt that you may feel after having *felt* revolted, would be helped with PINE, and it may be that a guilt-based desire to protect is indeed a form of compensation for the repulsion. A lot of parents feel inadequate, a feeling that may be associated with their reproductive capabilities – unable to produce a normal human being – or feeling inadequate in their ability to rear a child with such special needs. ELM would help those who feel the responsibility is overwhelming. However, most parents who have been delivered of healthy babies feel inadequate, and it is quite usual to underestimate one's ability when faced with rearing *any* child. LARCH may also be of help because it is the remedy to restore confidence and belief in oneself.

Parents' long term behaviour towards a handicapped child may take several different directions Some reject the child outright. There are others who lavish an extraordinary amount of care, and those who become over-protective.

There is no right way or wrong way to react – we cannot help the way we feel – and so what is right for one family may not be right for another. We have all seen handicapped children, teenagers and adults out with a parent or guardian. We may admire a family who care for their handicapped child, and are therefore witness to the kind-heartedness, love and caring that can exist. Thoughts of how well other people seem to cope however, can become implanted in our own minds where they stand out as an example of the way we too should behave. Even after several months or years have elapsed, you may become locked into a battle with your conscience – a conscience that has been created by the example set by someone who is totally different from you, someone who has a different temperament and outlook altogether. Understandably, some parents may feel under pressure from society, and duty bound to care for a child whom they are unable to love, but as Dr. Bach has said time and time again, you have to do what is right for *you* – not what other people think is "proper".

Come what may, having given birth to a severely handicapped

infant, and when faced with the awesome reality of what lies ahead, what to do for the best is not an easy decision to make – if in fact you believe you have a choice at all – and ultimately it is not only a decision about what you want to do, but what is best for your child and other members of the family as well. Once again, guilt can raise its head and wave an accusing finger at you. PINE therefore would be helpful. SCLERANTHUS would also help you in your distressing dilemma, and WHITE CHESTNUT would help to ease the constant, haunting mental chatter. ROCK WATER would help those who feel an enormous sense of duty which may mean self-sacrifice against their will. Rock Water helps to ease the rigid thoughts that are fundamental in people of this nature. RED CHESTNUT would help those whose genuine concern for the child's welfare causes anxiety, fear and concern which is out of proportion, creating a great deal of emotional restlessness, or conversely, CHICORY if a sense of being "needed" is gratifying and causes a desire to be over-protective.

Outside influences also play an important part in a family's attitude. What will other people think? Will they hate us if we choose to put the child into care? Will they avoid us if we decide to bring the child up ourselves? Will they be embarrassed? Does the handicap show – perhaps they will not notice…? These are a few of the questions and thoughts that may run through the mind. They are all significant because they are real-life problems, dealing with real attitudes, and human nature being what it is, people often find it difficult to be impartial. If you are strong-willed and believe in what you are doing, then this is not likely to cause a problem, because you will be comforted by knowing that whatever you have chosen to do was for the right reasons. However, not everyone has such clarity of thought. For some, the emotional repercussions can be extremely harsh. Doubt, depression, self-condemnation, bitterness, guilt and so on, may then force their way back into the thoughts. GENTIAN is the remedy to help ease the doubt and give you encouragement; SWEET CHESTNUT for the "locked in" depression, as though there is no way out of the situation – the desperation which can often surround so many families in this position; CRAB APPLE for the self-condemnation and detestation of oneself; WILLOW for the bitterness; PINE for the guilt.

Sometimes it is not only one's emotions that suffer. Any problem in a family or between a couple can potentially put a strain on the marriage or partnership because we tend to take our frustrations out on those we care most about. Support of one another is important to you all, because it is ultimately left to you as individuals to find your own way, the way that suits you. Listen to your heart, say what you feel, hug your partner and reassure your children, and with the remedies to help you cope, you will come through it feeling at least relieved of pent up emotions, and gradually a more positive frame of mind will be with you.

Dr. Bach believed that life here on earth is but a single part of our *actual* life. He believed that True Life was that of our spirit, soul or Higher Self, and that during the course of that life, we have to learn about everything – emotional disharmony, pain, suffering, love, peace, war – and everything that happens to us during the course of our life, is for a purpose, to benefit our spiritual development and act as another step towards perfection which is ultimately what Life seeks to achieve for itself. If we consider the whole "handicap" issue in a spiritual light, then the trauma of the child, its parents and other members of the family is for a definite purpose. It may be the lesson that particular child or parent has to experience at that moment in their evolution. That is why there is no right or wrong way to tackle it, because each one of us has to do what is right for us personally, and although guilt, indifference, bitterness or heartache may be difficult to overcome and may make you feel terribly inadequate or wicked, even these emotions have a purpose. They are experiences, and it is by confronting them and overcoming them that you will be able to put the lesson behind you. Some people say that it is all very well taking remedies for this mood and that mood – indeed, every emotion that is described has a "Bach Remedy" answer to it! but they cannot make the child better; they cannot make the handicap go away. It is this hopelessness (GORSE) that causes people to give up or not be motivated enough to even try the remedies in the first place. But it is sad that people sometimes deny themselves the chance of feeling happier within themselves, and it is sad that they may discard the means to do it because the therapy is based so much on simplicity. It is sad because although we all know that the remedies are not going to miraculously alter the pattern our life has chosen, those who are not coping with this delicate situation are nevertheless hoping for a return of happiness and laughter, even just for a little peace of mind, and it is this that the remedies can help to achieve. All we have to do is reach out for them and let them help us help ourselves.

THE NEEDS OF THE CHILD

There are numerous forms of physical and mental difficulties, each with common signs and symptoms and each with particular manifestations, but children are children, no matter what form their suffering might take or what label has been attached to it. As far as the Bach Remedies are concerned, the emotional outlook is the important factor, not the condition itself, so the disability needs to be put to one side whilst the mood and personality of the individual child is considered.

Nevertheless, it does help to understand the condition as well because then our appreciation of the child's needs will be more complete. It would be impossible to consider every condition in this book, so I will look at some of the more common conditions and difficulties. The role the remedies play in each case, however, can be adapted to suit the needs of *any* child suffering with *any* condition.

CEREBRAL PALSY

This is frequently referred to or known as "spasticity", but there are varying degrees of severity, ranging from disjointed movements and defective growth to loss of feeling and disorientation. In most cases, it is the result of a birth injury but in some cases no cause can be established. Hyperactivity and unexplained aggressiveness are common associated symptoms and some of these children may also suffer with epilepsy. The most common form of cerebral palsy is associated with hemiplegia (paralysis of one side of the body) and this is bound to cause delayed motor development although the child should achieve milestones, albeit slowly. Learning difficulties may arise but speech is not usually affected and normal schooling can take place.

A most distressing type of palsy affects the whole body which writhes when attempting voluntary movements. There may therefore be feeding problems and speech difficulties due to disturbed co-ordination, but whilst there are some who may be affected mentally as well, these children, despite their gross physical disability, have normal intelligence. Frequently they are assumed to be mentally subnormal because their physical appearance, involuntary movements and speech difficulties give the impression of mental retardation. Yet, with the right stimulation and educational assistance, they can attain an IQ equal to, if not higher than, a "normal" child. As greater understanding of this condition and awareness of the child's normal intelligence has developed, the care and support that they receive has improved considerably, but there was a time when these children were merely left to vegetate in an asylum and given no opportunity to exercise their minds. Understandably, one of the biggest emotional problems they face is frustration. Frustration with being trapped inside a body that does not work properly, frustration because people who do not know them treat them like morons, and frustration at not being able to contribute to the learning process – joining in discussions, asking questions, voicing an opinion or conveying a lack of understanding for example. This frustration would have been several times greater in children who were cut off from society and labelled "insane". Thankfully those days of ignorance have passed, or at least they *should* have done because there is no excuse, with the knowledge that is now available, for such appalling treatment.

Frustration has a lot to answer for, giving rise to behavioural problems such as temper tantrums, which are a sign of frustration in any child, but exaggerated in these particular children. The Bach Remedies, although not intended as a treatment for the condition, can nevertheless help the child deal with the frustration and other emotions that compound the difficulties they already face. The choice of remedies depends on how an individual child reacts. For example, frustration may give rise to a fiery quick temper, irritation and annoyance with other people who seem to interfere or get in the way. IMPATIENS would be the remedy to choose for the type of child who responds in this way. Generally, the frustration may be helped with VERVAIN because this remedy helps to ease the tension associated with the desire to solve a problem but being physically unable to accomplish the task. A child who is unable to make people understand what he wants and as a result gets worked up into an inner frenzy would also be helped with Vervain. For the child who goes rigid or who is unbending emotionally, ROCK WATER would help. CHERRY PLUM is another remedy which is often appropriate because it is the remedy for those who fear for their sanity, or who feel they are going to "explode" – a feeling that frequently presents itself alongside frustration. In such cases the remedy helps to re-establish self-control. If however, the frustration presents itself as aggression and forcefulness, then VINE would be the remedy to choose. A combination of Vine and Cherry Plum would help children who fight hysterically. Some children become spiteful which again may be as a result of frustration, and would indicate HOLLY. Other children withdraw into themselves and are not outwardly demonstrative at all. If they daydream or seem to be "miles away" mentally, then CLEMATIS would be called for, or WILD ROSE if they are apathetic, lack enthusiasm and motivation. HORNBEAM would also be helpful if the child appears weary or lethargic. Some children find an answer to their frustration by demanding attention of others, and show off or become unruly. VINE would help those of a rebellious nature who have a strong and dominant personality, but CHICORY would be for those who simply yearn for attention and thus may become manipulative. HEATHER children have a similar effect, but in their case it is achieved by holding on verbally, making others listen by talking at them closely and intensely.

There are, of course, also children who try to hide the way they feel. They appear to be coping well, happy, content, but underneath it all, their anguish is great and may surface every now and then in a violent outburst. These children need AGRIMONY which may be a very helpful additional remedy to give in any case as they are all suffering inwardly and because no matter how extrovert they might appear to be, they are still locked inside a body that is unable to express what the normal active mind inside is trying so hard to do or say. Quite understandably, this anguish can lead to terrible bouts of depression for which SWEET CHESTNUT would be the most appropriate remedy because it is the despair and tortuous inner pain that causes such distress.

Another element which may be a problem for a lot of these children is fear. Fear of what will happen to them, fear of the people who are caring for them, fear of the people who teach them. Perhaps fear of pain and of being forced to do something that will hurt or which they know will be beyond their capabilities. Known fears require MIMULUS but if the fear is bordering on terror, which it may be from time to time, then ROCK ROSE would be appropriate on those occasions. If however, the child appears to be frightened or apprehensive, but it is not obvious exactly why he is afraid, then ASPEN would be helpful as it is the remedy for vague fears that haunt the mind for no apparent reason.

For times of great distress, panic, sudden alarm and other emergencies, RESCUE REMEDY would be helpful as it deals with all these elements.

❈ DOWNS SYNDROME

There are a variety of chromosomal abnormalities giving rise to a number of syndromes, but the most common is Downs, also known as mongolism.

The cells of a normal human being each contain 23 pairs of chromosomes, 46 in total. Chromosomes are the bearers of genes which make us what we are, each pair having a different function, from determining the colour of our eyes to whether we develop as male or female. In Downs syndrome, there is an extra chromosome so the baby is born with 47 in each cell instead of 46.

Downs syndrome children have similar facial features but the personality of each child will differ, as with all children. They do however, have many characteristics in common. For example, they are usually affectionate, become agitated when others are in distress, and enjoy imitative play. Generally, they are happy and friendly children and although their developmental progress may be slow, they will respond to and gain great benefit from stimulating play and learning opportunities, and can reach surprisingly high levels of competence.

Although I constantly emphasise the need to choose remedies on an individual basis and *never* to generalise, the positive aspects of

CHICORY (the remedy for those who have a lot of love to give, like to mother and are concerned for others), sums up many of the qualities of these children. Although at times, like everyone else, Downs syndrome children can be in a bad mood and then display the negative traits of the Chicory character – possessiveness, self-pity and selfishness – on the whole, they are content and balanced. Because they are usually of a gentle nature, they may be easily dominated, in which case CENTAURY would be a useful remedy as this would help them to gain sufficient strength to stand up for themselves, and also CERATO for those who are easily led and persuaded because they naturally want to copy and mimic. WALNUT would be helpful as this offers protection against outside influences. WILD ROSE may also be appropriate, as it is for those who are happy with life the way it is and go about daily routine with an attitude of complacent acceptance.

There will be times, just as there are in any other child's life, when temper, sulkiness and withdrawal are displayed from time to time. WILLOW would help with the sulky moods which result in sullenness and stubbornness. HOLLY would help the temper if it is directed at others in a spiteful, hateful or angry way. CHERRYPLUM if the temper is out of control. Another element which may be noticed is daydreaminess or distant thought. CLEMATIS would be the appropriate remedy in this case.

Although there are varying degrees of mental retardation amongst Downs syndrome children, they are generally very rewarding to care for. Their affectionate nature makes them responsive to kindliness and love, and they can be great fun to be with.

BLINDNESS

A child who is born blind will obviously not know what sight is, and so, although sighted people may be appalled at how disorientated, frightened or unfulfilled a blind person's life might be, to the person who has never known sight, it is not necessarily a problem at all. On the contrary, in many cases, enjoyment of food and music for example, can be much more rewarding because the senses of taste, touch, smell and hearing are heightened to compensate for the blindness. The palate for example is more sensitive and so appreciation of delicate tastes is greater. Indeed, if we are tasting something pleasant, how often do we close our eyes to enjoy it even more? Similarly, hearing becomes more finely tuned to intricate sounds – blind people learn how to really *listen* to things, rather than just hear them. Touch also becomes so much more interesting, and given an object to hold, the blind child will really explore it, feel it, touch it, imagining all the time what it is like. After all, one does not have to actually see in order to imagine, and the imagination of blind children can be even more pronounced *because* they are blind – their *mind* has to see in place of their eyes. Blind children therefore build up a world of their own. What they see in their thoughts, and how they imagine people and objects, may not actually resemble our own visual images, but that does not matter because the child is still relating to the imaginary images as well as the taste, sound and feel of things around him just the same. Blind babies, for example, will know their mother's voice, her smell and the feel of her face and body, and thus come to recognise her as well as any sighted child who has a visual image to relate to. Blind children will enjoy hard toys, things that they can feel and associate a shape in their imagination. It is really a matter of modifying the educational process in order to give them the stimulation they need to reach full potential and be able to learn as much as they would if they had been born with normal vision. Different skills will have to be acquired – learning to read Braille for example, or learning from the spoken word, recordings and so on. Although schools now have much better provisions for children with various difficulties, and there is much emphasis on integration, schools with specialist teachers and equipment specifically designed for the blind would generally be more appropriate, because the entire teaching programme would be adapted to cater for their needs.

With regard to the emotional outlook, children who have never known sight may not be distressed because they cannot see, but at times may wonder what it is like, and this may give rise to despondency or sadness because of their inability to experience it. Whatever other remedies they might need from time to time to help them cope with the normal emotional difficulties that any child would face, there are certain remedies that would be helpful to consider should the child feel left out or downhearted for these particular reasons. GENTIAN would ease the despondency and help to relieve a depressed state of mind; WILLOW if they should feel resentful towards sighted children or life in general; SWEET CHESTNUT if they feel a deep sense of sad despair; what they long for being out of reach. This may occur if they are constantly reminded of their sightlessness, or if other children make fun of their disability. CLEMATIS would be appropriate for children who drift into a make believe, imaginary world and thus may become distanced from the real world around them.

Children who have become blind as a result of an accident or illness, may also need some of the remedies mentioned above. It is understandable that they too may feel resentful at times, or unhappy. They may also feel frightened, especially at first and so MIMULUS would help to ease the fear and nervousness they are likely to feel. RESCUE REMEDY would be appropriate initially because it contains **Star of Bethlehem** to ease the shock, as well as **Rock Rose** for terrifying panic. Enforced blindness may also have an impact on children's overall emotional development. It may cause them to lose confidence in themselves for example, and in this case, LARCH would help them to regain the certainty they once had. They may also feel very lonely and cut off from the life and friends they knew so well. This type of loneliness is a form of grieving, for the loss of familiarity, the loss of eyesight. It is this sadness that causes the feeling of isolation. STAR OF BETHLEHEM would help the grief, but also WATER VIOLET if the child is normally reserved but now feels even more estranged from family and friends. WALNUT would be another useful and very helpful remedy, because a tremendous amount of adjustment has to take place and the change that the child has to cope with is dramatic. Walnut helps to make the transitional period a little easier by helping the child cope with such a different way of life.

For those who become so attached to the memories of the past that they dwell on the things they could relate to before they lost their sight, HONEYSUCKLE would help. The remedy will not delete these memories from their minds or make them forget what people, places and objects look like for these are important recollections which they will want to cherish for the rest of their lives, but if they have become locked into yesterday at the expense of today and tomorrow, then Honeysuckle is there to help them realise that the present is as important as the past.

❀ DEAFNESS

As with the blind, deaf children need to acquire different learning skills. The emphasis in learning will be on visual imagery, reading, writing and drawing. Deafness does not interfere with play as such, but a very deaf child will not have the opportunity to learn about sounds, which may make certain experiences difficult to comprehend. A cup or plate or other fragile object for example, will make a "crash" and break into lots of pieces if it is dropped, and because of this association between sight and sound, even when we do not see the object breaking, we know it is broken because of the sound it has made.

Learning about music and the environmental sounds of traffic, doors, water pouring, the waves at the seaside, animal noises and bird songs will, to a certain extent (depending on the severity of the deafness), need to be imagined, just as a blind child has to imagine what something might look like. With deafness however, watching a dog barking or a bird singing or seeing a door closing does not offer many clues and so it may be very hard to appreciate the concept of sound. Deaf children can, however, learn to appreciate music through vibration – touching the instrument and feeling the vibrational difference between one note and the next. Similarly, they can learn to play musical instruments by distinguishing vibrations. Beethoven of course, is a perfect example of just how *well* a deaf person can perform musically.

Deaf children, as they learn to read and write, have to modify their learning in order to translate the spoken word into language they can use to communicate. Lip reading and sign language replaces sound with a form of non-vocal verbal shorthand, and these are skills a deaf child will need to learn.

One of the greatest problems faced by deaf children, is the effect their deafness has on their own speech. A baby with normal hearing would gradually realise that he is actually making the sounds he hears, and so will make them again and again, delighting in this new ability. Other sounds follow, and gradually they are compared to those made by other people, the baby begins to imitate the shapes formed by the talking mouth, and tries to copy the sounds he hears. This is the beginning of language, and even before the child has learned how to pronounce words properly, he or she will talk in a language that is thought to be understandable, regardless of whether anyone else can understand what is said! Constantly hearing words spoken and relating them to meaning helps children build up language skills and thus learn to talk, communicate and be understood. If a child is unable to hear what sounds he is making, then he is not able to modify his speech. This does not only apply to pronunciation, but also to the accent that is put on certain words, the "song" that goes into sentence construction, and the interpretation of what is said through the given emphasis. Deaf children can learn to speak by making a solid sound into words simply by making shapes with the tongue and mouth, and learning how to project the voice, but it is the intricacy of the language – the vacillation of the voice etc. – that puts emotion into it. Deaf children therefore, often seem to talk very flatly although vocal intonation can be learned with care and attention and special training. Thankfully *total* deafness is rare, and if the deafness is diagnosed early, the child, even as a baby, can be fitted with an appropriate hearing aid. Progress can then take place normally, and language and speech will have the chance to mature and become established during the course of development.

Some children cope with their deafness and the reactions of other children very well, but *any* child that stands out from the rest may risk being mocked. Loneliness, frustration, annoyance, anger and hurt are among the emotions that may be experienced, but appropriate remedies can help the child to feel more comfortable and able to cope with the attitudes of other children. For example, MIMULUS would help the child who is nervous, shy, timid or afraid; LARCH for the child who has little self-confidence; CENTAURY for the child who is bullied, taken advantage of or dominated by more confident, forceful children; VERVAIN for the frustration; GENTIAN for the discouraged child; WILLOW for the unhappy one; AGRIMONY for the child who hides his feelings; CLEMATIS for the child who seems to be in a world of his own; WALNUT to help protect and provide a shell against outside influence. This remedy would also help the child who has become deaf, due to trauma or disease, to adjust and cope with the upheaval it will inevitably have made to the quality of his life. As with the child who has become blind as a result of an accident, the child who has become deaf in this way is also likely to be afraid and panicky at first, and so ROCK ROSE for the terror, STAR OF BETHLEHEM (or Rescue Remedy) for the shock, and MIMULUS for fear, nervousness and lack of courage, would help to cushion the impact of such traumatic consequences.

Children who are coping with a disability can be much stronger than many adults in a similar situation. They tend to accept things better and are able to adapt to a new way of life much more easily, never ceasing to amaze us with their resilience and fighting spirit – perhaps budding OAK personalities. With the remedies to help them remain strong and positive emotionally, and given the right tools with which to learn, then whatever the *disability* might be, it need not become a *handicap*.

CHAPTER 7

Puberty

PHYSICAL AND EMOTIONAL CHANGES

Adolescence is, essentially, the transitional period between childhood and adulthood, beginning with the onset of puberty and ending with maturity. How long this actually takes varies from one person to another, but usually takes place over the course of several years. It is the chapter in life that is notorious for its turbulence and "problems" – a period of struggle and strife as the child and adult within the same individual meet.

Not only are there enormous physical changes taking place, but also psychological development and growing awareness, and young people have to cope with many strange feelings as they get to know their new body. Doubt and confusion seem to plague young people, and are responsible for a great deal of teenage unhappiness. Doubts about who they are, what they are, and whether they have a body that allows them to be the person they want to be. If they do not know the answer to these questions, then despondency and desperation can soon set in. There are two remedies that are ideal for these confusing issues: CERATO would help those who seek confirmation from others and need to be reassured that they are worthy, and SCLERANTHUS for those who are upset by choice, swing from mood to mood, and take on first one identity and then another, unable to choose which really fits them. Scleranthus helps them to stabilise their thoughts and to know where they truly belong.

Puberty signals the beginning of a series of changes as a girl becomes a woman, and as a boy becomes a man. The reason for this maturation is life's desire for survival and reproduction. The changes that take place in puberty therefore – the essential differences between children and adults – are sexual, so it signifies the stage of development when the secondary sex characteristics appear. The onset in girls occurs around the age of 11 or 12, although it may arrive sooner or later. Everyone is different. Boys tend to reach puberty a little later – at about 13 or 14, but again, each one is different. The developmental time-lag however, continues to be apparent throughout adolescence, girls maturing, on the whole, at an earlier age than boys.

In boys the physical changes that take place are mostly external and mainly visual and audible. The growth of facial hair, deepening voice, stronger jaw-line etc., as well as the gradual development of body hair, and of course, development of the sexual organs – an enlarging penis and yet more hair at the base of the abdomen and around the genitalia.

In girls, the changes are more internalised with the commencement of menstruation, but also the development of breasts and the growth of pubic and underarm hair.

In addition to these obvious physical changes, there are many other aspects of developing maturity that also cause a great deal of upset and disruption, and these are shared by boys and girls alike – spots, sweating and body odour for example. There is also a mountain of emotional surges that inevitably cause havoc mentally. A girl's swelling chest or a boy's squeaky breaking voice can cause acute embarrassment and so the Bach Remedies can play an important role in offering a helping hand to curb the anxiety.

❀ GIRLS

Menstruation

The menstrual period is central to a girl's pubescent development. It is, however, the result of a complex series of changes that begin some time before there is even a hint of the period actually starting. These changes are the result of hormonal activity, culminating in a regular monthly cycle, with menstruation occurring, on average every 28 days, although as with everything, each girl is different and so the cycle may be shorter or longer than this.

It is at the beginning and end of a woman's reproductive life when disruption to the rhythm of the menstrual cycle is most likely to occur. Sometimes following the commencement of menstruation, the periods do not appear again for a few months. Sometimes the cycle is so irregular that bleeding occurs anything from fortnightly to two-monthly, but usually the pattern settles down after a while. There is nothing abnormal about an irregular cycle during puberty, but if it should continue for longer than one might reasonably expect, then it would be wise to see your family doctor who will be able to set your mind at rest. There are some girls who mature physically – i.e. their breasts develop, they grow pubic hair etc. – yet their periods do not begin. This is not necessarily abnormal, as we all develop at a different rate. Eventually menstruation will more than likely begin spontaneously, but if a girl should reach the age of about 16 without having had a period, then once again, it would be wise to speak to your doctor who will be able to initiate some preliminary investigations if necessary and provide you with re-assurance.

Delayed or irregular menstruation however, can cause a great deal of stress and this itself tends to antagonise the smooth running of this delicately balanced cycle. Hormones are very susceptible and easily influenced by stress and the cycle can be disrupted to such an extent that the periods may stop altogether. Because the remedies are for the relief of stress, they can have an *indirect* bearing on the cycle if its disruption is due to emotional upset. WHITE CHESTNUT, for example, would help to relieve worry; MIMULUS would ease the fear caused by what *might* be wrong; WALNUT for the adjustment to the changes taking place; AGRIMONY for the girl who tells no-one about her worries and pretends all is well, yet suffers inner agonies that she does her best to conceal.

Delayed menstruation may be very worrying indeed. Thoughts like "where does the blood go?" or fears that noxious substances – all the waste from the body have been left inside. The remedies as mentioned above would help to ease the fear and worry, but the addition of CRAB APPLE would also be helpful as this is the cleansing remedy and will help those who feel that to *not* have a period is unclean and so have a desire to get rid of something and expel it from the body. Menstruation, however, is not a waste disposal system, and there is no storage of blood inside the uterus if a period fails to arrive.

The first menstrual period, when it begins, can be quite a shocking experience, no matter how well the girl has been prepared, for until it actually happens she will not know exactly what to expect. Girls who have *not* been prepared adequately, such as those who have not received any sex education and do not know anything about periods and reproduction, may be terrified that they are bleeding to death or that at the very least, there must be something horribly wrong with them. Schools are getting better at providing sex education, but frequently it comes too late, after the event, and it therefore rests with parents to explain the facts of life to their children. The parents' attitude towards personal matters will naturally be reflected in their approach to the subject. If they are shy and extremely reserved about anything to do with sex, then their embarrassment may be transferred to their daughter who may regard sex as unpleasant and her periods as dirty. Or, for one reason or another, she may not feel she can talk to them about the subject, so her questions remain unanswered, her fears and apprehension deepen, and as she seeks advice from friends, may be misinformed. Be this as it may, we cannot help the way we feel, and if something makes us feel awkward, then no matter how hard we try, we are not going to be entirely relaxed about it. Parents are naturally concerned for their children and so although they may *want* to explain the facts of life to them, when they find that they *can't*, feel terribly guilty for not having provided them with the information they need. The harder you try, the worse it becomes – your daughter knows you feel uptight and *you* know that she knows how you feel, so you are *both* conscious of the situation which adds to the awkwardness and makes you both as embarrassed as each other!

Come what may, periods and all that goes with them can indeed be difficult. Menstruation is, however, a completely natural process and nothing a girl should feel ashamed of. If she is able to talk to someone – mother, sister, aunt – who is able and willing to offer a straightforward explanation of what it is all about, and how to handle it when the time arrives, this will go a long way towards easing the fear and awkwardness so frequently experienced.

When the periods do start, each girl will react differently – some may be blasé, others panic stricken. Some may want to tell everyone and consider it an exciting moment, whilst others will do everything in their power to keep it a secret. The remedies for each girl there-fore, will be different. For the girl who is afraid, MIMULUS would help ease her nervousness. It is also for girls who are shy or self-conscious due to their changing body and sense of vulnerability. ASPEN is a useful remedy for the panicky fear of the unknown, or at least the unknown element surrounding the object of the fear. ROCK ROSE would help the girl who is absolutely terrified – or perhaps terrified at the sight of blood. This remedy may be especially relevant for the girl who is unprepared and does not know what to expect, does not know that she is supposed to bleed. Naturally, under these circumstances, it will be a great shock, for which STAR OF BETHLEHEM would be required, along with Rock Rose for terror, and CHERRY PLUM for hysteria. These three remedies are contained in RESCUE REMEDY which may therefore be just as, if not more, appropriate in this instance. For the girl who cannot bear the state that her body is in, cannot bear the bleeding and feels dirty because of it, CRAB APPLE would help her to feel more comfortable with herself, *like* her body and appreciate that periods mean that she is becoming a woman and that in itself is something to be proud of. AGRIMONY is an important remedy for girls who try to hide the bleeding, do not tell anyone and pretend nothing has happened.

Apart from the initial shock and other emotions that accompany the beginning of menstruation, there is also the more practical side of its management to consider. Sanitary towels, fortunately, are becoming more and more comfortable. At one time, girls had to wear huge wads of cotton wool that bulged through their pants so that everyone knew they had a period, especially during physical education at school which could be a living nightmare. They made you walk as though you were wearing a nappy, were difficult to dispose of and had to be held in place by an uncompromising form of suspender belt! Before that, girls had to put up with pieces of material and anything else they could find that would be suitably absorbent. It is no wonder that periods became known as "the curse"! Today, sanitary pads are self-adhesive, slim yet highly absorbent, and much more comfortable to wear. They come wrapped in neat little packets so are no problem to carry to school and thus avoid the inevitable embarrassment of huge sanitary towels protruding from the school bag. Some pads are thicker for extra protection during heavy days, but even the thick ones are thin compared with their cumbersome counterparts that young women had to put up with in years gone by.

Tampons are not generally recommended for a very young girl, mainly because of the difficulty experienced in actually inserting them. It can be very painful and may well cause more problems than it solves. After a while, however, she may become more and more motivated to use internal protection. The first time may be so difficult that it puts her off altogether or she may feel very nervous about trying again, afraid of the pain, that she will damage herself or that she will bleed even more. If she feels like this, then it would be better for her to wait a little longer and try again when she is a bit older by which time she will be more physically mature which should make it much easier for her. There are, however, remedies to help ease the mental tension, in particular RESCUE REMEDY for the shock, terror, panic and feeling of faintness that accompany a bad experience; MIMULUS for the fear of pain or damage; OAK for the girl who struggles on despite everything until she has mastered it; ROCK WATER for the girl who *forces* herself to use the tampon, and even though it hurts her and she hates it, *makes* herself continue. In this instance, CRAB APPLE may be appropriate as well because it may be the dislike of "dirty" pads that is the driving force.

PERIOD PAIN (dysmenorrhoea) is another symptom of menstruation that can be equally, if not more, troublesome than the bleeding itself. It is common but varies in severity from one cycle to the next and from one woman to the next. The cramping pain usually begins sometime during the 12–24 hours before the period actually starts, and usually only lasts for 24–48 hours. It may cause faintness and nausea, and the pain, together with all the other symptoms, can be very distressing. The ideal remedy is RESCUE REMEDY because it contains **Star of Bethlehem** which helps to relieve the shock to the system, **Rock Rose** for the great fear attached to such terrific pain, **Cherry Plum** for the panic, **Clematis** for the faintness, and **Impatiens** for the annoyance and impatience that causes tension and worsens the pain. It may also help, as well as taking the Rescue Remedy orally (4 drops in a glass of water or juice), to apply it externally – a flannel soaked in warm water to which a few drops of Rescue Remedy have been added, and then placed over the lower abdomen can be very comforting. Drops of the remedy can also be added to bath water (about 10 drops or so) and this too can be very soothing. OLIVE would also be helpful because the endurance of pain can be exhausting.

PRE-MENSTRUAL TENSION, the emotional disturbance prior to a period, also poses problems for a lot of girls and women, causing irritability, depression, annoyance, temper and so on, and in extreme cases can almost bring about a complete personality change! WALNUT is the remedy which will generally help to re-establish balance and enable the system to settle down to a smoother rhythm, but for the emotional symptoms of pre-menstrual tension, remedies such as IMPATIENS for irritability and impatience, BEECH for annoyance and intolerance, MUSTARD for the depression, HOLLY for the temper, CHERRY PLUM for uncontrollable rage, and CRAB APPLE for the bloated, ugly feeling, are indicated.

Breasts and Bras

Wearing a bra for the first time is a strange experience. Not only is it uncomfortable but it is also an embarrassing item of clothing to have to expose. Bra straps have a habit of dropping off the shoulder and hanging out from under a short sleeved shirt. Their shape can be identified through clothing and so can their whole outline if you happen to wear a black one under a white blouse by mistake! Nothing seems to conceal the fact that a girl is wearing a bra, and if she is the only one in her class who *does* need to wear one, she may soon find herself being pointed at and talked about which, naturally, will not do her confidence any good and only adds to the multitude of emotions she is already having to cope with. Because of the uncertainty faced by most girls of this age, it is important to them to feel they belong. No one wants to be the odd one out, but the uncertainty may lead to despair and consequently cause a girl to become lonely and unhappy. At the other extreme, the girl who is the *last* in her class to wear a bra, may find the tables turn when *she* is the odd one out and the new victim of the other girls' mockery.

The same problems are often faced by those who are too thin, too fat, too well-groomed, too unkempt, too spotty... But whatever the reasons for the sarcasm, the feeling is the same, and the remedies are given for the feeling not the situation. Some of the remedies already mentioned in this chapter may be of assistance, but most commonly perhaps: CRAB APPLE for self-dislike, and for feeling the need to cover up and hide her body because she feels it is an object of personal shame; SWEET CHESTNUT for the despair and anguish that makes the way things are seem as though they will never change; WHITE CHESTNUT for the mental arguments that circulate in the mind; WILLOW for resentment towards other girls; LARCH to restore confidence; CENTAURY to help her stand up for herself and not let the other girls' remarks and banishment get the better of her, WATER VIOLET for the loneliness, feeling cut off or isolated, particularly if the girl is of a reserved nature anyway.

Breasts, of course, come in a variety of shapes and sizes. Even an individual pair are not identical. There is no "right" size – every woman is different. Some have large breasts, some have very small ones. What we are endowed with, however, does not always make us happy. Girls who are naturally buxom often wish they had small rounded breasts, and likewise, girls who are "flat" chested may long to have large voluptuous ones. I don't suppose anyone would have *pendulous* breasts by choice, but we can't have everything!

Whilst there are those who are not satisfied with their figure, feel ashamed of it, want to hide it, or get depressed over it, there are others who are very proud of their attributes and have no hang-ups whatsoever. Most girls fall somewhere between the two – reasonably happy but a little self-conscious all the same.

❀ BOYS

Because the pubescent changes taking place in girls are so obvious, and the associated difficulties so well documented, it is often assumed that boys sail through puberty with hardly a backward glance. Some boys probably do, but for others it can be just as, if not more, traumatic than for the average girl.

The physical changes that take place are the result of production of the hormone testosterone. It stimulates the development of the penis, prostate gland etc., and also causes the growth of pubic, under-arm and facial hair, the larynx to enlarge, thus deepening the voice, development of muscle, bone structure, and so on. The size of flexed muscles, broadness of shoulders and other physical attributes often enduce a competitive instinct amongst boys. For a boy of small build, this may well become a period of discomfort as he is whispered about or giggled at for being "puny". Naturally, this influence is likely to destroy a great deal of his self-esteem and make him feel very self-conscious.

Boys are therefore often under pressure to live up to a "macho" image, and if they are not as tough as the stereotype portrays, then they are frequently accused of being "sissies" which is guaranteed to shatter their confidence in one blow! Boys who are regarded as sissies are usually those who are reluctant to join in with certain pranks or who decline from doing something dangerous or playing somewhere that will make their clothes dirty. Boys who have female friends are often name-called sissies and may be accused of playing with dolls, or something equally "girlie". Boys who make a fuss about being home in time for their dinner may also be told they are sissies or accused or being "mummy's boy". Whereas some boys can take it all in their stride and not let it get to them, feeling quietly confident in what they do, other boys feel desperately uncomfortable and become depressed, nervous and tearful as a result.

Sadly the emotion that an upset boy shows as a result will provide the other children with even more ammunition because crying is probably the strongest evidence of "sissiness" that boys could wish to see! The "boys don't cry" injunction that is impressed upon men by society puts boys under a great deal of pressure when it comes to feeling strong emotion. They are, after all, no less capable of feeling tearful, compassionate or hurt than women, yet society generally seems to accept female tears but scorns at a weeping man. There is therefore, pressure on boys to keep their emotion to themselves, to be hard not soft, to be tough not weak, dominant not submissive. Yet not all boys are of the same nature. There are as many gentle, peace loving and humble boys as there are extrovert, anything-for-a-laugh, rough and ready types, yet the conventional male is the epitome of this macho image – something which portrays only a handful of men in reality. So what is wrong with a boy showing his feelings? What is wrong with wanting to be helpful? The answer of course, is absolutely nothing – they are good, fine qualities, but sadly the male ego seems to try and suppress that gentleness at times. Perhaps that is why men are referred to as "gentlemen" because most of them *are* soft-hearted underneath.

Remedies to help boys who are struggling to live up to the expected role image, depend on how they respond to it. If they lose their confidence, LARCH would be helpful. If they are easily dominated, pushed around and have trouble standing up for themselves, then CENTAURY would be their remedy, and it is unfortunate that because of this gentle nature, they can become easy prey for others to make fun of. Boys who become introspective, dwell on how miserable they feel and are tearful with resentment, WILLOW would be the remedy to lift their spirits. MIMULUS would help the boy who is shy and nervous and may lack the courage to fight back. CHICORY would help the boy who needs to be loved, wanted, accepted, and begins to cling as a result – clinging to his peers, even those who call him names, hanging around them, wanting to be their friend, and clinging to parents for comfort and attention. Chicory is the remedy for those who, in effect, love too much and because of the way they react when they feel snubbed, suffocate the very people they want to be close to. HEATHER would help the boy who becomes overly talkative, possessive in a verbal way, becomes obsessed with himself and tries to portray a better image by boasting about his attributes, his new bicycle, the amount of pocket-money he receives etc., thereby hoping to win approval. Heather people feel lonely when they have no friends around them, and so Heather children, adolescents and teenagers feel even more lonely if they are outcast.

On the other hand, there are those who, despite remarks from others, remain cool and collected, and brush them aside as though they really did not matter. Those who genuinely take it in their stride in this way would be OAK personalities, and the remedy would help them to regain their strength should that inner driving force begin to weaken. If, however, the boy *seems* to be outwardly brave and confident, and instead of withdrawing into himself or shying away from other boys, becomes a form of clown, making others laugh, excelling himself by entertaining as a means of diverting attention away from his apparent shortcomings... and if underneath the bright and breezy exterior lies an anxious, worried and depressed soul, then the remedy AGRIMONY would help to relieve all that torture and help him to feel more relaxed.

BODY ODOUR

As the body wakes up to advancing adulthood, part of the maturing process is the development of the hair follicles under the arms and in the pubic area. As the hair follicles develop, so the pores and sweat glands are activated. It is this activity that causes sweating, especially under the arms, and if not checked, will create "body odour". Never during childhood will a girl or boy ever have needed or even thought about deodorant or anti-perspirant, and so they may only first become aware of their body odour and active sweat glands when a friend mentions that they smell "sweaty". Again, acute embarrassment may be a problem, and a growing paranoia about smell may develop. CRAB APPLE is an extremely valuable remedy because it would help those who feel uncomfortable with themselves to appreciate what is happening and calmly put it right, instead of allowing it to become a reason for self-hatred. After all, if we get worked up about the fact that we are sweating, we will sweat even more and so it can become a vicious circle, creating deepening discomfort. Crab Apple would also help those who become totally obsessed with hygiene, *constantly* washing and being over-anxious about smells and sweat. In addition, MIMULUS would help those who are fearful, to have more courage to face others, and LARCH would help those who have lost their confidence.

Some children are extremely good and conscientious when it comes to washing and keeping themselves clean, but most children tend to skimp a little – just wash what they have to, quickly, which usually means only the face and not the other areas of the body that also need attention. I wonder how many times "have you washed your neck?" has been asked, and how many children have honestly been able to say "yes"! Puberty, therefore, is a time when washing and daily hygiene routine needs to be put into practice for real. It becomes increasingly important as adolescence progresses but it can take time to get used to the idea. In the meantime, therefore, it may require constant "nagging" to drive home the importance of keeping oneself clean and fresh. As girls and boys get older they realise for themselves how important it is, and then it will be difficult to get them out of the bathroom at all!

III | **SPOTS** | Sebaceous glands, particularly prominent in the skin of the face and scalp, produce an oily substance called sebum which drains into the hair follicles and reaches the surface of the skin as the hair grows. On the skin's surface, its positive attributes keep the hair soft and shiny, provide the skin with a certain amount of water resistance and act as a bactericide, protecting the skin from the invasion of harmful bacteria. Sebum also acts as a lubricant and prevents the skin from drying and flaking in the open air, sunshine and hot dry atmosphere. Its negative aspect occurs when the follicle becomes "clogged up" with sebum causing a blockage. This plug of sebum then becomes infected by micro-organisms in the air, and by transferring bacteria as one touches the face. The infected follicle causes a lump under the skin to form (a pimple), often with a white or black visible head. Some spots are large but have no head and due to the pressure of their presence in the skin, cause pain. All spots are formed this way and so all spots are, in effect, acne, although the condition of acne as a skin disease by and large excuses the very mild eruption of spots and concentrates instead on severe cases. Usually, adolescent acne disappears by early adulthood, but if it is very severe, it may persist for longer and could result in scarring.

Acne vulgaris, to give it its full name, is an understandably troublesome complaint. There is always a temptation to squeeze or pick the spot to release the sebum. It is, however, advisable to try and resist the urge because it may introduce more bacteria (thus more infection) and a worsening of the condition in the long run. There is also a danger from persistent squeezing, of damaging the skin itself, and leaving permanent marks on the face which will only become another source of distress later on. Washing with a mild soap and water daily, keeping hair clean by washing it as soon as it begins to feel greasy, perhaps three or four times each week, and wearing it so that it does not aggravate the face, will all help to deter bacteria, avoid infection and thereby reduce the severity of the condition generally.

A number of sufferers have found the application of CRAB APPLE extremely helpful. Simply add a few drops to sufficient clean water to rinse the face, or better still, add 2 drops to an egg-cup full of water and dab the solution onto the affected areas with cotton wool.

If this is done morning and night after washing, the remedy will have a chance to really help. The use of creams is not usually recommended for sufferers of acne, on the basis that the skin is oily enough already. This, however, is not an entirely accurate assumption. If the skin is *clean* – i.e. it is washed regularly, then adding a moisturising agent will not necessarily introduce bacteria and should not therefore have any harmful effects, although some skin types are, nonetheless, sensitive to creams, lotions and moisturisers of any kind. The RESCUE REMEDY CREAM is a bland salve that does not contain lanolin. The base contains honey and other natural ingredients to which **Rescue Remedy and Crab Apple** have been added, making it a very versatile, soothing and healing salve. It has proved to be helpful in cases of spots and acne, but again, its application should be when the skin has been cleaned. Applied at night, the remedies in the cream will be able to get to work, so a good night-time skin cleansing routine could involve (1) wash, (2) rinsing or dabbing with Crab Apple lotion, followed by (3) the application of the Rescue Cream to individual lesions, gently massaging it in with a clean finger. This routine may need to be followed religiously for a while, but if improvement is taking place it will instil confidence and encouragement to continue.

In addition to the physical discomfort of the condition, there is the emotional aspect to consider. The name "acne vulgaris" has a rather off-putting ring to it to begin with! The name itself suggests that it is vulgar, unpleasant, sickening and so it is not surprising that it is regarded in such a way. Sufferers certainly may become extremely self-conscious about their appearance and begin to despise themselves. CRAB APPLE is again an important remedy as it helps them feel more comfortable with themselves, and would be a useful remedy to take *anyway* for its cleansing properties.

The emotional side-kicks from this condition can be enormous. Not only the feeling of self-disgust, but the inhibition and self-consciousness it can cause are just some of the states of mind experienced by adolescents trying their best to cope with all aspects of their body image. Despite the fact that it is a problem shared by the majority of adolescents, albeit in varying degrees, this knowledge is usually of little solace to a severe sufferer. In addition to Crab Apple therefore, LARCH (for confidence) and GENTIAN (for the feeling of dismay) may also be appropriate.

Depression can set in for some adolescents and there is a mixture of reasons for this. The hormonal disturbances stirred up by the onset of puberty, together with the growth of self-awareness and search for identity, are all possible causes of depression, but add to this a badly blemished skin, loss of self-worth and sense of rejection, the depression may easily become utter despair. SWEET CHESTNUT is the remedy to help relieve this desperate anguish and deep unhappiness. GORSE would help to revive hope and optimism, and WILLOW to look outside oneself and realise the happier side of life is still there.

Acne can cause skin irritation as well as pain, and this may also create irritation in the mind. IMPATIENS is helpful for this feeling. Impatiens would also help those who feel impatient if their spots seem to take a long time to heal.

IV THE DESIRE TO BE THIN

Body image is a prime concern throughout puberty and adolescence, and is not only related to what we *actually* look like, but more importantly, what we *want* to look like and what we *think* we look like. We may compare ourselves with others and covet the looks of someone else, perhaps feeling dowdy in comparison and wishing we had more dress sense or colour co-ordination, or a different shape to carry clothes better. How we look to others and how we feel about ourselves is important at any age, but it is especially important to the image conscious teenager who is only just beginning to make an impression on the world at large, and who wants to be liked, attractive and sought after.

Very few adolescents are satisfied with the way they are – they may feel their facial features are not attractive, that their legs are of the wrong shape, that their hair is the wrong colour, too frizzy or too straight, that they are too tall or too small, too stocky or too lanky. In their attempt to improve their looks, girls and boys may become obsessive about their physical appearance and can both go to extraordinary lengths in order to achieve the sort of image they want. Girls may embark on serious dieting to acquire a trim figure, but boys too have hang-ups about their shape, size and features, and so although extreme slimming was at one time considered to be a female activity, there are more and more boys who are now also starving themselves to lose excess weight and look good. This is often combined with a rigorous exercise regime designed to build muscles, but because physical activities like this require a lot of energy, weight loss can be too rapid and result in physical and mental fatigue if the food intake is not sufficient. As a result, there may be a danger of the teenager becoming anorexic.

Anorexia nervosa is the tragic illness where sufferers hardly eat anything, and starve themselves because of their desire to be thin. It can get to the stage where they see themselves as fat and ugly even when they might be flesh and bone. It is a most unhappy condition and anyone who has an eating disorder needs a great deal of help and support.

There is frequently a degree of self-dislike and a great amount of doubt and uncertainty about their worthiness, but there is usually an underlying cause as to why they should have such poor self-respect – perhaps they have felt that they have not been praised sufficiently and so do not have very much confidence, or maybe they have been told on repeated occasions that they are fat. There may be a problem with a relationship – family, friends boy/girl friends – which causes them to punish themselves this way. They might feel guilty about something and feel they *deserve* to be punished, or they may do it out of resentment or spite. Clearly it is important to ascertain the cause because then the most appropriate remedy can be given. The following are some which may be particularly helpful:

SELF HATRED – CRAB APPLE – for the self-dislike and detestation. It is for a sense of ugliness and grossness and self-condemnation. It is also for the abhorrence of food, feeling that it is dirty and will contaminate the system. Bulimia is the sister disease in which the sufferer has periods of bingeing, vomiting and then intense dieting. With this disease, the self-dislike aspect is apparent just as it is with anorexia nervosa. The Crab Apple remedy helps sufferers to know, respect and accept themselves for what they are.

SELF SACRIFICE – ROCK WATER – this remedy helps to ease the tension and rigidity associated with self-denial; when people force themselves to stick rigidly to a diet or train themselves so harshly that they have to vomit or starve. Rock Water people reprimand themselves for being weak and thrive on a self-punishing regime that denies them even simple pleasures. The state of mind may be generated by self-hatred (CRAB APPLE), or associated with feelings of guilt (PINE), or it may stand alone as a type remedy in its own right. Rock Water also helps those who have had the hard taskmaster attitude ingrained upon them by the self-righteousness of people around them. Whatever the cause of this frame of mind, the remedy helps the sufferer relax and be less harsh, and accept that life is not about sacrifice and deprivation, but that there is give and take, pleasure as well as pain.

GUILT – PINE – this would help to ease a guilty conscience or guilt complex about something a person thinks he or she has done. It is for those who blame themselves and believe that they are the cause of whatever goes wrong. The remedy will help them to put those guilty feelings out of their mind or at least into perspective, so they can accept that they are not to blame for everything.

CONSTANCY – WALNUT – this remedy will provide protection from outside influences, and the disturbing effects that others may have on the natural flow of one's own life. Walnut helps to shield the person from these influences so that they are able to pursue their own calling and progress in their own way, free of the interference of others.

ANIMOSITY – WILLOW – this will help to overcome feelings of resentment or bitterness, self pity and introspection that may be the reason why teenagers punish themselves – the "I'll show them" attitude. Unfortunately it is *they* who become the victims. Willow will help those who feel this way to be more optimistic about their life generally, help them to forgive what they blame others for, and help them to cast their thoughts in a more open and outward direction so they begin to concentrate on issues other than themselves.

DOUBT – ELM – this would help those who feel unable to cope with life, overwhelmed with the responsibility of approaching adulthood, the sexual changes taking place, or with the array of new emotions and experiences as they grow up.

UNCERTAINTY – CERATO – this would help those who feel insecure and desperately need to be reassured that their life is worthwhile, and that they have a valuable contribution to make, thus helping them realise, and believe in, the quality of their existence.

FEAR – MIMULUS – this remedy is for fear and would therefore help those who are afraid of being overweight, or afraid of eating in case they should put on an ounce of weight. Unfortunately the fear of over-eating exacerbates the problem. They are afraid that food will harm them and so their diet becomes progressively limited, generating a deepening fear of eating. The resulting emaciation caused by such an extreme habit can cause yet more fear, but also utter exhaustion (OLIVE), resignation (WILD ROSE), and loss of hope (GORSE).

If a teenager is genuinely overweight and wants to do something about it, then he or she will need help, reassurance and encouragement to do so safely. Obesity is not healthy and can be a recipe for a miserable existence, so a positive approach to a sensible weight loss programme is the first step to a better self-image generally. However, adolescence is a period of growth and so the body needs to have quite a high calorie intake. It needs a well-balanced and sustaining diet. A teenager's "reducing diet" therefore is not one that demands unusual eating habits. On the contrary, the diet should be normal, because obesity is caused (in most instances) by over-indulgence in the *wrong* kinds of foods – primarily those which contain sugar. By cutting out these unnecessary fattening foods, weight control can be achieved safely and healthily without depriving the system of important nutrients or necessary calories.

Remedies that would be helpful are those such as GENTIAN to provide encouragement; CRAB APPLE to promote better self-image; CENTAURY to prevent the teenager becoming a slave to food; HORNBEAM to give strength to face the new eating regime; IMPATIENS for the sense of urgency and impatience to be thin quickly. If progress seems too slow, it can cause a lot of people to give up. Impatiens therefore, promotes patience.

GORSE would help any loss of hope or a pessimistic outlook that nothing is going to work, SWEET CHESTNUT would help to relieve the helplessness and despair that so many people feel when they are reminded of their weight problem, and WALNUT, being the link-breaking remedy, will help them adapt to a new way of living, step out of the way they were, and overcome past habits. If history keeps repeating itself, CHESTNUT BUD will offer insight to break the chain reaction that might be responsible for weight gain a second or third time around, having forgotten why it happened in the first place and how miserable it was.

V	**THE DISABLED ADOLESCENT**

When we consider all the hang-ups that normal able bodied adolescents have, they seem so trivial when compared to what a disabled adolescent has to put up with, for not only do they have to worry about things like spots and hair colour, but they have the added burden of the disability itself.

Disabled children and youths, however, seem to develop a tremendous strength which helps them to overcome some of the things that may otherwise stand in their way of self-love and acceptance. They often have to put up with a lot of unpleasant remarks, being made fun of, talked about, laughed at and so on. They need to be strong and often they are. They may be OAK personalities if they are genuinely brave, or AGRIMONY types if the bravery is a façade. Nevertheless, there are bound to be moments of unhappiness, anxiety, fretfulness, despondency and despair.

The remedy for despondency or depression *because* of something in particular, perhaps negative thoughts about their handicap and how it will affect their ability to lead a normal life, is GENTIAN, or GORSE if the despondency is a morbid hopelessness. SWEET CHESTNUT would help those who feel utterly trapped and unable to see a way out of their difficult situation, feeling so helpless and forlorn, to see a little light on the horizon. Sometimes it is those who pretend to be cheerful (Agrimony people) who eventually succumb to the Sweet Chestnut state because they hide their anxieties and feelings so much that they suffer inwardly, unable to share their grief with anyone, and so it has no escape. Eventually that inner pain turns to anguish and if that is the case, then a combination of both Agrimony *and* Sweet Chestnut would be appropriate.

Disabled adolescents may face other difficulties too – meeting people, gaining entry to certain places, having to rely on someone else to take them and bring them home again. It is this dependence on others and lack of autonomy that can be the cause of many emotional difficulties – guilt (PINE), self-condemnation and disgust (CRAB APPLE), self-reprimand, self-punishment (ROCK WATER), despondency (GENTIAN), despair (SWEET CHESTNUT), or it may cause them to go to the other extreme and actually *enjoy* the attention they receive (CHICORY). Those of a very strong-willed and determined nature may dominate the people they are dependent upon (VINE), may feel sorry for themselves, and resent others for being able-bodied (WILLOW), become aggressive (VINE for dominant aggression, or HOLLY for an angry, spiteful, revengeful or hateful aggression), or completely apathetic, drifting through life, accepting what does or does not come their way, content with what they accept as their "lot" in life (WILD ROSE).

Society as a whole often seems to ignore the needs of the disabled – many places are not equipped to cater for their requirements which means that they are prevented from enjoying certain activities or leading a normal unrestricted life, simply because they are the minority and an able-bodied society has not considered their needs with enough planning. The sexual needs of the disabled are also often disregarded, pushed into a corner as something un-important or unnecessary, yet their sexual needs are no different to those of the able-bodied. If a person breaks a leg he becomes dis-abled for a while, but just because he cannot move freely does not mean that he no longer has any interest in sex. Similarly, for those with a permanent disability – they have the same needs, and the same rights. Sex education for handicapped children and adolescents therefore is just as important as it is for any other children. Every-one needs to understand the messages they receive, the impulses and urges and the unusual things that might occur as a result of those feelings. To remain ignorant can lead to fear and confusion and create a complicated layer of discomfort. But careful attention to their needs and help for parents to understand their needs too, will go a long way towards establishing a sense of belonging within the school community and society generally.

CHAPTER 8

Love, Sex and Sexuality

SEXUAL IDENTITY Sexuality and sex are two quite different subjects yet frequently considered as one and the same. Sex refers to gender or to the physical act of sex. Sexuality, on the other hand, has to do with how we feel about ourselves, how proud we are of our respective bodies, and our sexual identity.

The development of sexuality begins at birth when gender is established and development as a male or female begins. Many parents are very conscious of not wanting to establish role models and make a concerted effort to dress their children in unisex clothing, buy unisex toys and so on. But it is difficult to be completely impartial and inevitably boys tend to be predominantly given boats, trains and cars, and girls dolls and shopping trolleys. Nevertheless, children *like* to play "let's pretend" and act out role models by imitating their parents. Left to their own devices, however, without the influence of traditional male/female role conditioning, they will join in any activity. Girls would probably be just as interested in a car's engine if they were consistently invited to help dad in the garage, and boys would be just as interested in cooking if they were encouraged to help mum in the kitchen (or vice versa – some mums are better with cars, some dads are better at preparing the dinner!). If girls and boys have the opportunity to be involved in everything, they really would be independent when they grow up. This might be easier in theory than in practice, but the way we *expect* children to behave and thus sometimes subconsciously, plan their activities, must, without doubt, have a bearing on their own role identity.

Society too places pressure on the growing teenager, imposing demands which they may find hard to cope with. The media can make it difficult for adolescents to grow up at their own pace because

149

sexuality is often forced upon them, and as a result they are made to become aware of their identity before they are ready. If this occurs too prematurely, it will cause even more uncertainty, and then sexuality *is* in danger of being confused with sex and sexual freedom.

II | SEXUAL IMPULSES

The development of sexuality occurs as a result of natural curiosity. At about the age of 5 months, a baby discovers his toes and, like everything else, they find their way into the mouth. This is how the baby explores and finds pleasure – the mouth, after all, is a sensitive area which is why eating and kissing are so pleasurable. Once a baby begins to find his toes, hands, feet… he will naturally begin to explore other parts of his body too. One often sees baby boys and toddlers tugging or fiddling with their penis. This does not mean that they are masturbating, but simply that they have discovered something else to play with and are learning about it. There will, however, come a time when they will realise that it gives pleasure, and even a very young child can have an erection. This is quite normal, and is really only another developmental milestone, which of course they will all come to sooner or later, although it might take the child – and the parents – a little by surprise.

In boys, the hormone testosterone is responsible for the adult sexual urges, and although as children, they may gain some infantile pleasure from handling their genitalia, it is not until puberty that they actually sense physical sexual impulses and arousal.

Virtually all boys, and men come to that, will experience the ejaculation of semen during sleep (often referred to as a "wet dream"). It may be spontaneous or the result of an erotic dream. It is normal but may take place repeatedly and can be worrying to a number of boys, especially if they do not know what it is. They may become embarrassed about the stain on the sheets, worry about having to sleep at a friend's or relative's house in case they make a mess. They may feel desperately ashamed, feel they must be dirty or abnormal in some way and then become too embarrassed to talk to anyone about it and so do not receive the reassurance and explanation they so desperately need. Boys who have been brought up to understand that sex is rude and have been discouraged from having girl-friends, are those who are most likely to be disturbed and upset by nocturnal ejaculation. It is therefore important to prepare them by explaining simply how their body works and why, and about the facts of life. This will help to allay their fears and help them feel more comfortable about discussing their feelings and asking questions about sex.

Similarly, boys who have derived pleasure from fondling their genitals, may be suddenly surprised when semen is first emitted. Again preparation as to the body's function so they understand what is going on when it *does* happen, is important. However, although masturbation is natural, and only an extension of the self-learning process, it can, in some instances, become a compulsion and a socially unacceptable obsession. Boys who become so absorbed may well have other emotional difficulties besides, and once these are settled, their sexual behaviour returns to normal. Psychotherapy can be helpful, but the remedies may, of course, be used alongside. Obviously, the important aspect to consider first of all, is the *reason* for the behaviour – whether there has been a disruption in his usual routine, such as a family crisis, bereavement, divorce of parents etc., a big change or upheaval such as moving house or school, difficulties associated with friendship or an unhappy relationship with a teacher for example – and the appropriate remedy can be chosen for the way the boy has reacted to such an occurrence. For any shock, sadness or sorrow STAR OF BETHLEHEM would be helpful. For any change or upheaval, WALNUT is the required remedy, and it will also act as a link-breaker to help resolve the habit. For fear, MIMULUS (for everyday nervousness) or ROCK ROSE (for terror) are remedies to consider. In addition to this, it is important to establish the boy's personality and temperament generally and choose a remedy appropriate to his personal needs. Then, we need to consider his feelings with regard to the obsessive masturbating itself, *why* he needs to do it, how he views it etc., and select remedies to help him overcome any negativity that he may be experiencing. CRAB APPLE would help to ease the compulsiveness, but would also be appropriate if he should feel a sense of disgust; PINE if he should feel guilty; VERVAIN if he does it to overcome frustration and tension; perhaps he feels strongly about something but cannot do anything about it...; VINE if he is aggressive and this is his way of releasing that aggression; CHERRY PLUM if he is unable to exercise self-control; CENTAURY if he has become a slave to it.

Some boys can become very distressed about it – they want to stop, but are unable to. They can feel desperately unhappy, afraid there is something terribly wrong with them and become frightened and worried as a result. GENTIAN would lift their spirits and help them feel more positive, MIMULUS would help relieve their fears, or ASPEN if they do not know what they are afraid of yet are filled with a strange feeling of apprehension or unexplained excitement.

This sort of behaviour does not only apply to boys of course – girls also explore their bodies and so may manifest masturbatory behaviour, and similar remedies may apply to them too, depending on their individual needs. Although girls cannot exactly have a "wet dream", they can certainly experience erotic dreams and may have an orgasmic response which wakes them up. They too may feel guilty, frightened or disgusted. It may prey on their mind, puzzled by what has happened, or worried that they might be a sexual freak. Reassurance and explanation about sex and sexuality will go a long way towards putting their minds at rest, but it is more helpful to prepare them before it happens than to wait until after the event, just as it is much easier to prevent the fear and shock of the sight of menstrual blood by gentle explanation beforehand than it is to try and allay the fears of a terrified girl who has already convinced herself that she is seriously ill.

When children reach puberty, the hormonal activity connected with their sexual development triggers sexual impulses which generate physical attraction between one person and another. Usually boys become attracted to girls and girls to boys, but sometimes homosexual or bi-sexual behaviour is apparent. This too can be a perfectly normal part of growing up, and most adolescents who indulge in some form of experimental sexual activity with a member of the same sex, grow up to lead perfectly normal heterosexual lives. The experimentation they might have indulged in during puberty or early teens, therefore, will have helped them to discover who they really are, and establish their true sexual identity.

Some adolescents may continue to be homosexually attracted and because they are in the minority, their feelings are frequently a deep source of concern. They may wonder what is wrong with them when their friends are swooning over magazines showing off scantily clad models, or talking about someone they fancy. Homosexual adolescents may not understand their feelings and so try to force themselves to join in with their friends' enthusiasm, yet all the time never really feel heartily involved. It can be a period of immense uncertainty, the adolescent becoming increasingly confused about sex, sexuality, their own personality and where they fit into it all.

It may only be transitory, but nevertheless, they may feel very lonely, ashamed or alienated, making their teenage years extremely uncomfortable. Remedies to help in this situation are SCLERANTHUS for the uncertainty, and not knowing which sexual role to adopt. CERATO would be for the lack of faith in themselves, the need for reassurance and confirmation, although this may come later because at this initial stage, the adolescent may feel too confused to ask for advice, perhaps hoping that if they do not mention it, it will all go away, and one day they will wake up, as if from a dream, and be "normal" after all. For those who try their best to hide their feelings, put on an act and pretend that they are having fun like everyone else, when in actual fact they are going through inner torture, AGRIMONY is the remedy required. CRAB APPLE will help those who feel ashamed of their feelings. LARCH will help those who do not have the confidence in themselves to stand up to the pressures of society. MIMULUS is for courage; WATER VIOLET for the lonely alienation; CHERRY PLUM if they are afraid they are losing their mind or that they are mentally sick; WALNUT for protection and to help break the link with the ties that may be preventing them stepping forward; CERATO for those who are easily led, adopting the identity of a role model and going along with an idea because they are unsure about what they really want; CENTAURY for those who are easily controlled or dominated, and PINE for those who feel terribly guilty.

Most adolescents, however, are attracted to the opposite sex and so once a girl begins to take on a more womanly figure, boys will naturally become aware and attracted. Because boys' development in adolescence comes later than girls', it is usually older boys that begin showing an interest.

This can, understandably, be unnerving for the young girl, although the reaction is bound to vary considerably. Those who are self assured and full of confidence, will be able to rise above it and handle the situation as they wish to. For a girl who is not so strong willed, or does not have as much confidence, it can be quite worrying and traumatic. I have to admit, that I can clearly remember the first time it happened to me, and although in hindsight the whole incident was extremely trivial and innocent, at the time it seemed horrific. I was only about 12 years old at the time, and as I walked through the school to the next class, there were a group of four or five boys aged about 15. One of them cut across my path and said "I fancy you". That was all that happened, but it frightened and worried me desperately. I suppose I did not know what he really meant – did he want to rape me? I felt so confused that I didn't tell anyone for a long time, but eventually owned up to a teacher. When I opened my mouth to recite the incident, it sounded so silly, I'm sure the teacher must have wondered what on earth all the fuss was about! The incident itself, however, was a separate issue. Whatever it was that happened, or didn't happen in this case, the feelings were real enough.

Looking back, the remedies that I would have chosen are WHITE CHESTNUT for the worrying thoughts that I couldn't help from entering my mind, MIMULUS for my fear and nervousness and lack of courage to face the situation, STAR OF BETHLEHEM for the shock it gave me, perhaps ROCK ROSE for the nightmarish panic, CRAB APPLE for my acute embarrassment and sense of vulnerability, and AGRIMONY because I kept it all to myself, although once I had plucked up the courage to tell the teacher, suddenly everything was in perspective.

III FALLING IN LOVE

Developing a relationship with a boyfriend or girlfriend is very important for most teenagers. Overcoming the initial shyness of attraction and attention is a major hurdle when getting involved with someone of the opposite sex for the first time. First relationships may be clumsy and difficult to cope with. Being stuck for words, not knowing what to do, what to say, and being frightened about what might or might not develop, creates anxiety which does not pave the way for a particularly relaxed encounter!

All sorts of emotions go round in the mind of a young couple in this situation as each one struggles to show the other that they are experienced and know the ropes, and yet ironically, each is probably as naive as the other and equally desperate to overcome their own embarrassment. However, no-one is alone, and these hiccups in early relationships (and later ones) are natural and follow an entirely normal pattern. There are, of course, certain remedies that can help a young person to cope with their feelings:

MIMULUS – for the shyness, timidity and nervousness that are encountered by many boys and girls. Sometimes this is particularly helpful for boys who are generally expected to make the first move. They have to pluck up enough courage to ask a girl out, and face possible rejection, and fear of receiving a negative response may cause some boys to back out. Mimulus would help them to have the courage to seize the opportunity, make the move and, more than likely, be pleasantly surprised at the result. Mimulus will also help those who are shy, blush easily and may feel too embarrassed to approach a girl, simply because it makes them feel uncomfortable and afraid of looking a fool in front of her (and her friends).

LARCH would be a helpful additional remedy and often accompanies Mimulus because where there is lack of courage, there is often a lack of confidence too. Larch is the remedy to bring about a return of self-confidence, thus overcoming the fear of failure, and stimulating a firm belief that attempts *are* likely to succeed.

SCLERANTHUS – this remedy helps the emotional dilemma, the uncertainty and hesitancy that wastes time and energy and achieves very little, except frustration. Scleranthus helps those in such a state to be more decisive and convinced of what they really want to do, and then have the forthrightness to go ahead and do it.

Adolescents frequently idolise pop stars, actors and other well known figures. They also often develop crushes on school-teachers or older pupils, and become completely transfixed by the attraction that person stirs in them. In some it takes over their thoughts altogether so that they lose interest in other activities, school-work and friends and begin to withdraw from active home-life. Similarly, during the early stages, in the development of a boy/girl relationship, a "love-sickness" can develop, causing the young person, having fallen for someone (usually before the relationship has begun) to become mentally absorbed with nothing but thoughts and dreams of that person, imagining what it will be like to go out together, hold each other's hand, what the first kiss will be like etc. This imaginary world can certainly be enjoyable, but it can also be distracting and result in loss of concentration, excessive day-dreaming and absent-mindedness. CLEMATIS is the remedy to help the thoughts focus on what is happening *now*, so that adolescents enjoy and do not dream away their youth.

The teenage years may be considered to be a period during which young people are able to practise and experiment with relationships until they find the person with whom they want to share their life. Many young people have several boyfriends or girlfriends, falling in and out of love at regular intervals, until a serious relationship eventually develops. This may not necessarily be the relationship that lasts into adulthood, but it will certainly have a profound effect on the couple involved. Relationships formed at school can last for several years, but once experience of life is gained, it can mark the beginning of the end of that particular partnership. The end of a relationship is painful, and the end of a first love relationship is likely to be traumatic for *both* the young people involved. The trauma can be intense and the emotions exaggerated considerably because those involved are still new and raw, and like the young shoots of a plant are easily hurt and damaged.

The remedies can be of great help in soothing and healing the scars and because the anguish can be so pronounced, this may be the occasion during which the remedies are of most value during teenage years. Again it is the individual response that will determine the appropriate remedies for a specific person, but this selection covers the most common emotional difficulties:

DESPAIR – SWEET CHESTNUT is for the sense of utter devastation as though one's whole life has crumbled. The future looks desperately bleak and life no longer seems worthwhile. It is the remedy for anguish of the soul – heartbreak.

CHERRY PLUM – teenagers, because their feelings are so fragile, sometimes seem to over-react to situations, their emotions are heightened and their responses more extreme than an onlooker might think appropriate. For the teenagers themselves, however, it is no act, and the feelings they have are very real, so much so that they make rash decisions or become overwhelmed with a sudden compulsion to do some irreparable damage. Sometimes that damage might be towards themselves with an urge to commit suicide (see also Chapter Nine). Cherry Plum is the remedy to stabilise irrational thoughts and behaviour and helps to calm the mind before something regrettable happens. Usually the motive for attempting suicide in this situation is a reactionary emotion and done on the rebound in anger, panic or desperation. Cherry Plum would be helpful to give should this reaction be a known danger, or should the teenager display a hysterical mood, uncontrollable emotion or express fear of doing themselves some harm.

SORROW – STAR OF BETHLEHEM is primarily for shock and will therefore ease the sudden blow that news of the end of a relationship may cause. It also helps the trauma generally – the feeling of grief and sadness at having lost the loved one. It is the remedy that heals the wounds, soothes the heart and acts as a comforting and reassuring bridge across the emptiness.

MENTAL RESTLESSNESS – WHITE CHESTNUT would help those who find they are mulling the events, possibilities, whys and where-fores over and over, unable to rest or relax enough to obtain sufficiently refreshing sleep.

MEMORIES – HONEYSUCKLE is for the memories and thoughts of the past that overshadow any interest in the present. Honeysuckle is the remedy to help lift the thoughts back into the present day.

PESSIMISM – GORSE is for the outlook that makes everything seem negative. The remedy helps to turn the negativity into optimism, restoring belief in the future and life itself.

GUILT – PINE – it is quite common for teenagers to blame themselves for the break-up of a relationship, believing that it was their fault and wishing that they had not done a particular thing, or feel guilty because they had. The guilt can eat its way right into the person's core and cause them to carry the burden of guilt and self-blame around with them for a long, long time. Pine is the remedy to help free the mind of the pent up guilt and so release the weight of this destructive emotion.

VENGEANCE – HOLLY is to ease another highly destructive emotion – hatred. The hatred can cause a lot of anger and that anger can simmer within a person where it creates a desire for revenge, suspicion or jealousy of other people's relationships or the estranged partner's new boy/girlfriend. The Holly remedy helps to transform the angry hateful feelings into something warmer and more heart-felt, so as to help the love that had temporarily been snuffed out by the flame of hate, jealousy and anger, to return. WILLOW in addition to, or instead of Holly would also be useful as it would help those whose anger has become internalised, forming a deep grudge and sense of lingering bitterness.

IV

SEXUAL ACTIVITY & ADOLESCENT PREGNANCY

In previous generations it was accepted as normal routine and correct for a girl to meet, court and marry one man and to respect her virginity before marriage. It was probably unthinkable to have sex before marriage even with the man she was destined to marry. Marriage took place at a much earlier age than is average today and women accepted their role of housewife and mother and the majority probably never thought about a career of their own. It was a male dominated society and women accepted their place in it without question.

As the years went by, women began to see themselves as capable of contributing to society in their own right. This was the start of the social change and as it progressed, young people pursued their personal identity and happiness which led to marriage at a later age, pursuit of a career and equality. It also involved a need to express their sexuality as individuals and seek satisfaction through sexual fulfilment. This invariably involved more than one relationship and this new "permissive" society which had grown up so quickly was frowned upon by the generations it left behind.

With this change in social trend came the realisation that sex education was necessary and that young people should be more knowledgeable about their bodies and understand reproduction. However, despite apparently appropriate sex education, adolescent pregnancies continued to occur in alarming numbers, and this still provokes a number of questions: Are these pregnancies the result of ignorance? Should sex education be aimed more predominantly at the 9–12 year olds? Is sex a "dirty word" at home and are children's feelings about it confused with the different attitudes of parents and teachers? Do we teach too much or too little, and are we teaching the right things? Does it lead to experimentation without or in spite of sound knowledge and understanding of its effects? Do adolescents actually *have* sound knowledge and understanding?

Most young teenagers feel the need to conform within their peer groups and do not want to "lose face" with their friends by not being involved in the same activities. Talk about boyfriends will often arise and each will be quizzed about the intimacies of their relationship with questions like "how far did you go?" Some will give a detailed account which may often be purely fantasy rather than fact. This may lead to a more sensitive member of the group feeling that she is "missing out" and feeling that perhaps she *ought* to go further than she felt was right herself. This can, evidently, lead to disastrous consequences. It is not only female friends who can cause this pressure however. Boys are renowned for their detailed run-down of their sexual experiences and can often contribute to pressurising their girlfriends into "giving in" (albeit sometimes unintentionally). The girl may be faced with what she sees as the ultimate option of losing her virginity or losing her boyfriend, and at that age the heart invariably overpowers the mind and, as a result, the boyfriend wins.

Even with a sound understanding of the implications of intercourse and a sensible attitude towards the need for contraceptive precautions (especially in light of the dangers of contracting Aids and other sexually transmitted diseases), social pressures still arise. To carry condoms may not always be considered acceptable as it may suggest that the girl is anticipating intercourse which will place her in an awkward position when the time comes. She is perhaps more likely to present herself as unprepared rather than face the embarrassing situation of presenting her boyfriend with a contraceptive, and so the condom remains in the place where it is least effective – in her pocket!

No matter how disappointed parents might be at the thought of their daughter submitting to sex before marriage, or how much they might want to dissuade her from sex at all, let alone safe sex, the fact remains that young people *do* indulge in sex, and although some, as I have described, are pressurised into it, if a girl is in love with someone, then it is only natural that she will want to express that love in a physical way, and likewise for her boyfriend. It is therefore preferable that she should do so safely by protecting herself from not only pregnancy but from sexually transmitted diseases, but unless she has received adequate advice on contraception, she is likely to be careless. Part of sex education, therefore, may include advice on sexual precautions, and although many people view this as a means of encouraging teenage promiscuity, if adolescents are going to do it, then surely it is better for them to protect themselves than to become victims of ignorance. Contraceptive advice does not necessarily encourage sex – on the contrary, if the pitfalls are described lucidly enough, it will act as a deterrent, and at least it will provide young people with the information they really do need to have.

The first time is likely to be awkward, uncomfortable and messy. It may have taken place behind a bush, in the back of a car or in the garden shed, and even if it took place in the comfort of a bedroom, it was most probably shrouded in tension for fear of being interrupted. It may therefore have been a rushed, undignified, clumsy and unpleasant experience, causing numerous emotional feelings that serve to put it under an even bigger cloud. Guilt and shame (PINE), self-disgust and embarrassment (CRAB APPLE), disappointment at having been unable to say "no" (CENTAURY), at being easily led (CERATO and WALNUT), and depressed as a result (GENTIAN), filled with remorse and regretting every minute (HONEYSUCKLE). For a girl to find out a pregnancy has occurred *as well* is like applying a bitter icing to an already flat and tasteless cake, and needless to say, will create untold misery and agonising despair.

She may well have been in a state of panic during the couple of weeks following the event, anxiously awaiting her next period. If menstruation has only recently begun, it may not have yet established a regular cycle which simply adds to the stress of the situation. A less well informed girl or perhaps one whose periods have not yet started (but were just about to), may not even realise what might have happened and the pregnancy may therefore continue unnoticed until it is well established.

The fear of pregnancy can be so stressful that it is sometimes pushed to the back of the mind with a rather unstable self-reassurance that "if I forget all about it, it will go away". In many cases the girl will be too frightened to go for help (MIMULUS), fearing the response from her parents or doctor and of course this, to her, is disastrous. Most parents, after the initial shock (STAR OF BETHLEHEM), are usually understanding and just as worried about it themselves, and would therefore seek help for their daughter without delay. But if they don't know, they can't help. There are, sadly, some parents who will reject a girl in this position; some will refuse to have anything more to do with her. Her boyfriend may well be supportive, but some boys are "scared off" by the whole situation and shun their responsibilities by refusing to take any blame or denying the incident altogether. The young girl may then have to face the problem alone.

Whether her parents are behind her or not, she has to face the important and traumatic decision of what to do about it. She has three stark choices: (1) To continue with the pregnancy and keep the baby; (2) To continue with the pregnancy and have the baby adopted; (3) Have the pregnancy terminated.

If she decides to keep the pregnancy *and* the baby, she will need tremendous support and help from those around her, especially if she is very young. A 16 year old and her boyfriend may decide to marry, but this can lead to more stresses and strains for the young couple. Whether or not they are responsible and have a steady relationship, there is always the possibility of feeling dissatisfied (GENTIAN, WILD OAT), and resentful (WILLOW, HOLLY) as time goes on. After all, 16 is young and if they are a family at that age with the enormous responsibilities that brings with it, doubt and regret may soon creep in as youth slips away from them. They see their friends going out and having fun with no ties and this can lead to unhappiness and loneliness. There are, of course, some who cope extremely well, and growing up *with* children can be a lot of fun, but all the same, it is sad that they have missed out on independent adventure during what are probably the most important years of their life.

To continue with the pregnancy and have the baby adopted may seem a satisfactory answer if termination is not acceptable. This still presents its problems however. School-work will suffer, the girl will have to face her friends while she is pregnant which can provoke some sneering remarks at school, not to mention the physical traumas that pregnancy and childbirth carry, and the mental anguish of giving up the baby at the end of it all (STAR OF BETHLEHEM, SWEET CHESTNUT).

Termination therefore may seem the simplest way out, but even this is not problem-free. It is a traumatic experience and one which may stimulate emotions in a girl that she is unprepared for – guilt (PINE), shame and disgust (CRAB APPLE), shock and a sense of bereavement (STAR OF BETHLEHEM), nightmares, terror and panic (ROCK ROSE and CHERRY PLUM), deep regret (HONEYSUCKLE), fear (MIMULUS), bitterness (WILLOW), suspicion (HOLLY). The whole traumatic event may indeed leave the girl feeling bewildered (CLEMATIS), desolate (SWEET CHESTNUT) and emotionally scarred. The appropriate remedies, therefore, given when needed, can be a tremendous support to a girl in distress, and by helping her overcome the emotions encountered there and then, would help to reduce the possible repercussions.

❀ THE YOUNG FATHER

Although the young father may well shy away and deny it ever happened, some accept their responsibilities and want to be actively involved in whatever happens.

Many need to have their paternity acknowledged, and have the opportunity to discuss their feelings. The role the young father plays, however, is often limited by his immaturity as well as, on some occasions, his unwillingness or inability to bear the financial responsibility that may be involved. He also has to cope with other difficulties and constraints such as parental pressure, opinions, conflicting advice, disapproval, rejection by his school, and, in addition, if his girlfriend is under the age of consent, there may be fear of prosecution. At first a boy may simply lack the courage necessary to admit paternity, and he may run away from the situation because he feels guilty and helpless. When he does eventually accept his involvement and turns for help, he may find that everyone is too wrapped up in the stresses surrounding the pregnant girl to be concerned about the young father whose emotions are also in turmoil, and as a result, he becomes a rather nervous and unhappy onlooker.

The remedies are there to help him too, and those which may be particularly helpful are: MIMULUS to give him courage; PINE if he should feel guilty; ELM for the overwhelming sense of pressure and responsibility; CENTAURY to stand up and be counted and have his own needs taken notice of; AGRIMONY if he is pretending to be unconcerned, and WALNUT to help him adjust to the enormous change that has taken place in his young life.

CHAPTER 9

Social Behaviour in Adolescence

THE BEST WAY OF UNDERSTANDING adolescents is perhaps to look at our own youth and reflect upon how we behaved when we were their age, and what emotional struggles we experienced. I imagine most of us would remember a period of fraught relationships with parents, being cheeky, rebellious and so on. One memory may be of being reprimanded for doing wrong, yet unable to see any wrong in what you did. This conflict may be because as children we are led to believe that if we are told we are wrong, then we must be wrong and therefore accept it without question, but as we get older, we start to wonder whether this is in fact the case, and so a transformation from the childhood belief of "I'm *always* wrong" to the revised belief of "I'm *never* wrong" begins.

During this period, the adolescent is in limbo, neither a child nor an adult, and is vulnerable to the influence of everything going on around him. He becomes confused about almost everything, not least his own personal identity, and due to a growing need for independence and broadening of his individuality, there is often a rejection of those aspects of life that have been a constraint in the past, the aspects of life associated with childhood from which he is trying to break free. There develops a resistance to parental control or influence, even a rejection of their guidance, and the adolescent may no longer seek their approval or invite their company. Instead, he begins to conform and respond to peer group culture, something that plays a major role in adolescent sociability. However, because adolescents are vulnerable and exposed to a new world that they do not yet know or understand, they are in need of security and often find the comfort they are seeking by simply becoming one of the crowd. This may involve the adoption of idiosyncratic behaviour – dressing in similar fashions, wearing a similar hairstyle, talking in the same tongue, listening to the same type of music and so on. Ironically, therefore, in their quest for independence and freedom from conformity, they are, in effect, choosing to trade in one set of rules for another. This may be because they are still in the process of searching for their own identity and until they find it, they remain caught up in a cycle of insecurity and apprehension.

One of the most prominent writers on adolescent psychology is Erik Erikson who has termed the search for identity during adolescence an "identity crisis". This has become a well used term, and something that is almost *expected* of adolescents, frequently used to explain certain behaviour that manifests itself at this time. Because it has become, to a large extent, casually accepted as a normal aspect of growing up, the term itself may have turned full circle and actually become *itself* responsible for the so-called identity crisis. Even Erikson has wondered whether so many young people would be manifesting identity crises if they did not think they were supposed to! Do adolescents therefore behave the way they do simply because they are *expected* to behave that way? This question leads us to another, more fundamental, question – is adolescence really a problematic period at all? Do adolescents as individuals see themselves as going through a crisis or is it just that adults view it as a problem time because adolescent behaviour is different from adult behaviour? Certainly it is a period of awakening, exploration and soul-searching. It is a transitional period between childhood which is restricted in many ways, and adulthood when behaviour is again restricted by the conservative attitudes of society generally.

There will always be a school of thought that focuses on the extreme – drug addiction, delinquency, alienation and school-girl pregnancy – and makes an assumption that *all* adolescents experience these problems, that adolescents generally are a nuisance and a threat to the "calm adult dominated" society. Adolescence itself then becomes a "problem", but this conclusion is not altogether fair because so many of these so called adolescent difficulties are not confined solely to the young. Many adults experience drug addiction, alcoholism and unplanned pre-marital (or pre-permanent partnership) pregnancy. But is an alienated adult regarded as a threat to the community? Is it not more likely that alienation in adulthood is looked upon with sympathy, whereas an alienated adolescent is considered to be awkward, rebellious and an embarrassment to the family? Why is it that pre-marital sex in adulthood is (now) usually accepted, but pre-marital sex for a teenager is regarded with disapproval and disappointment? Young people are reaching maturity sooner now than they were in previous generations, and so it is not surprising that they feel frustrated at being treated like children.

During adolescence one is able to explore life and become expressive, and it is this expression that is often regarded as deviant by society at large. In their lust for adventure, fear and consideration of possible consequences rarely enter the mind – if it's fun, let's do it! Things that would turn one's stomach a decade later, do not even cause a flutter to an adolescent. They therefore often take risks – risks that the average adult would not dream of taking. Dare-devil feats and acrobatics fill them with exhilaration not fear, although even fear itself may be exhilarating. Being swept along with excitement and fun can make an adolescent seem thoughtless, selfish, careless and unruly, but this is usually a greater problem for onlooking parents who feel incapable of calming their apparently uncontrollable teenagers, than it is for the teenagers themselves. It is natural for adolescents to experiment with life and with themselves by trying out new fashions, hairstyles and so on. Some will also experiment with drink, drugs and sex in their quest to find out who they really are. Some simply want a taste of adulthood and a glimpse of what might be in store for them. For others, it may be a desire for adventure, to try out new things and experience what everything has to offer – after all, how do we know what is good and what is bad, pleasant and unpleasant, what hurts and what comforts, until we have actually tried things out for ourselves? As with everything in life, it is only through our own experience that we learn.

Some adolescents get involved in activities against their will, but because they do not want to appear to be the odd one out or regarded as a "goody goody", they will go along with the crowd just to prove that they are not weak. Ironically, it is those who say no and risk being outcast who have the most strength.

For those who are easily influenced or easily led, there are three remedies that would be of help – WALNUT for protection against outside influences, offering help to remain true to their own chosen direction, CERATO to help young people believe more strongly in their own convictions so that they do not have to prop themselves up by doing what the others do, but are able to be independent and certain that their judgement is correct, and CENTAURY for succumbing to control by other people, the remedy to give strength to say "no" and stand up for themselves.

For those who are on the other end of the scale – the ring-leaders of the group, the remedy indicated is VINE as this is for those who are strong-willed and have a tendency to dominate and take charge. BEECH may also be helpful as this remedy is for those who are critical of others, are unable to accept people for what they are, and instead get annoyed with their short-comings or make fun of their weaknesses. The remedy helps those of this nature to be more understanding.

TRUANCY, LYING AND STEALING

An underlying problem such as an emotional upset or difficult home life is usually regarded as being responsible for this type of behaviour. Certainly this is true for a number of adolescents, but it is not always the case. Some children stay away from school because they are being bullied or harrassed, or because their school work is too difficult and they do not want to face the subject. Sometimes truancy simply presents a more exciting option – the adolescent doesn't feel like going to school and so spends the day doing something else such as sitting by the river or wandering around the shops.

However, we should look at the reasons why some young people feel bored with school, and why they do not want to go. Boredom is a common problem amongst adolescents. They are developing a lot of artistic skills and creativity, so they tend to fantasize and imagine life differently. This is why many teenagers tend to over-react to stress, play-act and over-do their emotional feelings in front of their parents. In a way, it is an attention seeking device and so CHICORY would be helpful, but for the boredom and lack of interest in present day activities, CLEMATIS would be the most helpful remedy. WILD ROSE and WILD OAT may also help – Wild Rose for an apathetic attitude, drifting along unenthusiastically; Wild Oat for those who do not have a clear direction as to which way they are heading and so become disillusioned and bored as a result.

Some adolescents however, play truant as a means of rebellion; as a message to society that they are not willing to conform to its expectations and limitations. There is often a degree of resentment towards life, towards teachers, parents and other symbols of authority. WILLOW is the remedy for those who feel hard done by and resent being told what to do. HOLLY is the remedy for hatred and will help those who get in a temper, become spiteful and deliberately set out to hurt others – their parents usually! VINE would help those who are strong willed and aggressive, those who "know" and object to anyone in authority who tries to control them.

Lying and stealing are other ways of getting back at society, although sometimes it occurs subconsciously, when the adolescent "can't help it", or does not realise he or she is doing it. Lying or fibbing may be a way of gaining attention, especially if fabricated stories achieve results, but again, it is the *reason* for them in the first place that is important. If it is due to lack of attention, then CHICORY would help, or HEATHER for those who have become obsessed with their made up stories and draw people to them in order to win friendship and company. CHERRY PLUM would help those who *compulsively* tell untruths, unable to stop themselves, as though there is some driving force urging them to do it, and CRAB APPLE for the desire to rid themselves of the compulsion. Stealing may also become a compulsive habit, and very often the person concerned does not know why he does it, but subconsciously it is often a cry for help, an expression of his need for someone to take notice of him. Here again, CHICORY would be helpful, and WALNUT to break the habit.

Adolescents very often feel under pressure and sometimes their way of coping with that pressure is to deviate from the normal expectations of reasonable behaviour. For those who have difficulty coping, ELM is the remedy to help them feel more in control. Some have a very pessimistic attitude and give up on life, or school, because they cannot see any good or future in it. For them, GORSE would be a helpful remedy as this would restore their hope. Confusion is also a cause of this type of behaviour – the confusion over what is right and what is wrong – and for this state of mind SCLERANTHUS would be indicated, and WILD OAT for those who simply want something to do, having nothing else to aim for. Wild Oat gives more direction so that ambitions can be fulfilled.

SMOKING, DRINKING & DRUG TAKING

SMOKING

Smoking is often something that begins as a harmless experiment. People do it openly, and because adults and other role-models indulge, it is only natural for adolescents to want to try it too. If they have parents who smoke, it is likely to be accepted as normal behaviour, and of course if parents are smokers then temptation is there in the house and many will take advantage of the situation and help themselves to the odd cigarette when no-one is looking. In a sense, much of it is to do with mimicry, and watching others smoke encourages many teenagers to want to join in. If their friends feel the same, then they have moral support and they encourage each other.

There has been a great deal of publicity with regard to the harmful and antisocial aspects of smoking, and this has helped to put a lot of otherwise susceptible teenagers off the idea altogether. At one time, smoking was portrayed as sophisticated and grown-up, something that attracted the opposite sex. It was flaunted and advertised as a sign of maturity. Since greater awareness about the dangers of lung cancer and heart disease and the conclusive association with smoking tobacco, it is no longer portrayed in this light, but in some circles the image remains as a symbol of adulthood.

Education is crucial, so that at least the facts are known and made clear. If the teenager goes on to ignore the facts that they have been presented with, then at least they are making an informed choice. However, sometimes experimental beginnings lead to full addiction, and so even when they realise the dangers or discover for themselves that it is not a pleasant thing to do – that it gives them a cough, makes their breath and their clothes smell etc., – they are unable to just give it up at will. To their horror they find that they cannot do *without* a cigarette, and so the awful battle begins.

As far as the Bach Remedies are concerned, the remedy that is most helpful in breaking habits is WALNUT as this will assist the re-adjustment and transition whilst the withdrawal is in progress. CRAB APPLE is also helpful as a cleanser.

❀ ALCOHOL

A similar situation applies to alcohol. It is the experimentation with an adult activity, the experience of being drunk, and the desire to try for themselves what certain drinks and cocktails actually taste like, that is so appealing. This too can cause an eventual addiction in some cases, although usually getting drunk, being violently sick and suffering for 24–48 hours with an appalling hangover, is enough to put most people off!

There are health hazards associated with alcohol as well of course – liver sclerosis being one of the most damaging – and so education and awareness of the dangers are important too, although the media generally tend to portray the pleasures associated with drinking more than the misery.

Most teenagers will probably have been to a bar and obtained a drink before reaching the legal age, and sometimes it is just the thrill of doing something they shouldn't and getting away with it that is the main attraction. Going to see adult films and dressing up to look old enough to get into a night-club are other ways of doing adult things before being legally considered an adult. It can however, be humiliating when refused a drink at the bar, or refused access to the club altogether, especially after having spent the best part of the afternoon and evening getting prepared for it! Sometimes the humiliation will generate anger which may in turn make them even more determined to do the things that society says they cannot do.

❀ OTHER DRUGS

Having smoked cigarettes and experienced the feeling that is obtained from drinking alcohol, the next step may be to try cannabis. Smoking tobacco has a mild relaxing effect. Cannabis is similar but creates a greater sense of relaxation and well-being. Because of its mild tranquillizing effect, it relaxes the emotions, the taker becoming either very giggly, happy and talkative, or if already feeling upset or depressed, then emotional relaxation may exaggerate the depression or unhappiness. Whilst smoking cannabis does not automatically lead to harder drugs or addiction, having experimented with one drug, the temptation is there to try another, just as one would be interested in tasting different drinks. It is the harder drugs that are addictive – cocaine, heroin, crack etc. – and although one would not actively intend to become addicted, perhaps confidently passing a remark like "I can handle it, I'm strong enough not to get hooked", nevertheless, it happens.

More recently, it has become almost fashionable to take psycho-active amphetamines – "designer" drugs such as Ecstacy – which have a hypnotic and livening, energetic effect, and can therefore enhance the experience of certain types of music – fast, beaty and accompanied by colourful images. The music itself can be hypnotic, and it is not surprising that teenagers may be swept along with the whole experience and accept a drug that promises to make it even better.

There is, however, something else that is easy to get hold of, cheap, legal and effective, and that is glue. Solvents are extremely dangerous and addictive, but sadly abuse frequently takes place in secret, and parents do not even know. Sometimes it is too late by the time they do become aware. Some children and teenagers are encouraged by friends, or curiosity leads them to experiment. Others, however, use it as a means of escape, and once hooked, it can be very difficult to dissuade them. It is after all a cheap, hassle-free way of obtaining oblivion – so to hell with the consequences.

❧ ❧

For some teenagers taking drugs or consuming alcohol provides them with a false sense of happiness and a means of helping them forget their misery. Unfortunately it does not solve anything, but because a calming and relaxing effect is obtained which allows them to forget their troubles, at least for a while, it is not difficult to eventually become emotionally dependent and then addicted. It is a desperately sad state of affairs when a young teenager feels so depressed that he or she has to seek solace this way, but it is essential to unravel the reasons why it happens in order to select the most appropriate remedies. The effect on a particular individual and how he or she is reacting to it are important considerations. Very often, AGRIMONY would be a helpful remedy because this is for those who hide their worries, unhappiness and anxieties behind a cheerful façade, and if by taking drugs or drinking alcohol their mask of good cheer stays in place or provides them with a false sense of security, then Agrimony is the remedy required. It will help them come to terms with their feelings and realise that there is a better way of dealing with their problems than suppressing their emotions with a drug. SWEET CHESTNUT may also be a useful remedy, and often it is those who are of the Agrimony nature, and keep their emotional turmoil to themselves, who suffer with a deepening sense of despair, and having reached the point when there seems to be no way out, turn to the one form of comfort that at least makes them feel a little better. Sweet Chestnut, the remedy for this frame of mind, will help the sufferer to find the light at the end of the tunnel, and regain the desire to go after it. If, however, there is no apparent reason for the depression, MUSTARD would be the remedy to help lift the cloud of gloom.

For some teenagers, it is the pressure of school-work or of living up to expectations that causes them to feel they cannot cope. They begin to feel inadequate and despondent, and in their attempt to regain their confidence, may turn to drink or drugs. ELM is the remedy for those who feel overwhelmed in this way, under pressure and unable to cope. LARCH would also be helpful for the teenager who lacks confidence generally. Those who turn to alcohol or drugs to act as a form of support because they want to feel and act more confidently would find a mixture of Agrimony and Larch helpful, because once again, they are trying to hide their true feelings, and living by pretence which makes them feel even more of a failure and so a vicious circle begins to form. WALNUT is a valuable remedy when someone is withdrawing from an addiction or habit, but it also provides protection from disruptive outside influences that distract the person from following their own path in life and who may become involved in drugs unintentionally. CERATO would also help in this respect, particularly for those who feel insecure and need reassurance and acceptance that they are as important as anyone else; those who "follow the leader" to provide them with a sense of belonging. Cerato is the remedy to help lift the cloud of doubt so that they gain a greater belief in themselves as a valuable member of society in their own right.

There are of course, many other reasons, and these may stem from a restrictive childhood, feeling of rejection, being ignored, reminded of failings, constant reprimand, being blamed for everything, to name just a few, and there are several remedies to help in these situations too: WILLOW for example, would ease resentment and bitterness that may be felt towards family, and HOLLY for the suspicious, hateful or revengeful anger that may be apparent and aimed at authority generally, parents included; BEECH for intolerance and criticism, and the annoyance that is often felt when things do not go the way they want them to; STAR OF BETHLEHEM if there is a sense of loss or feeling of rejection. This is the comforting remedy and helps to heal the emotional scars that may have been caused by an upsetting childhood or adolescent experience. CHERRY PLUM would be helpful for the loss of control of the mind, violent rages etc., and CHESTNUT BUD would help them to learn from the experience of it all.

BACK CHAT, MOODINESS & REBELLION

Because adolescence is an in-between age, and a time when the scope of imagination and independence are broadening all the time, a great struggle goes on in the mind and this may cause a struggle within the family as well. Adolescents feel like adults, know what they want to do, yet are restricted by parents who still determine what time they should be in, where they can and cannot go and so on. A great deal of frustration and resentment can easily build up because on the one hand the adolescent is reprimanded for acting like a child, and on the other *treated* like a child when trying to take charge of his or her own life. The result is that adolescents feel misunderstood and become resentful or disobedient out of spite. If told to be in by 10, they will not come home until midnight. If told they cannot go to a concert or party, will go anyway.

Although not necessarily vocal, this kind of rebellious behaviour is a form of back-chat, but there is also the verbal version – cheeky

retorts and rude gestures. Really, it is a way of expressing independence and single-mindedness, but can nevertheless cause a
great deal of disharmony and stress to the family unit. Tempers flare
and a row begins. Frustrated parents may be tempted to slap their
cheeky teenager, but this just adds fuel to the fire and makes things
even worse, but if this kind of scene happens in public it can be
extremely humiliating! A lot of anger is generated which can lead
to a complete loss of control and hysterical behaviour. CHERRY
PLUM is the remedy to help bring about a calmer attitude and put
things back into perspective. HOLLY would also help the boiling
mood of anger and explosions of "I hate you!", and VERVAIN for
the strain and tension associated with frustration and the sense of
injustice of just about everything.

When we reflect on our own adolescence, I expect most of us can
recall feeling moody and bad-tempered on occasions. The memory
of this may well include being constantly shouted at for being lazy,
stubborn, rude... recalling how our parents never understood us,
that they just wanted to stifle our freedom... how we might have
slammed doors, beat our fists on the bed, ran away, stopped eating...
The list is endless, but every negative attitude is likely to be there
somewhere! There are numerous remedies that can help
adolescents (and their parents) get through these moody years.

The classic "moody" remedy is WILLOW because it is for the
negative whirlpool that drags one down into self-pity. It is for feelings of resentment and occurs as a result of a difficulty in accepting
the card life has dealt, asking "why me?" and "what have I done to
deserve this?" In adolescence, this feeling is very common because
it is during this period of life when the adolescent focuses everything
on the self, and so creates a feeling of being picked on, put down
and blamed for everything. The result is a bad-tempered miserable
adolescent who walks around carrying a huge chip on his shoulder.
The mood does not always last long, usually it comes and goes, but
it is one that is fairly inevitable at one time or another. Visually, someone in the Willow state will frown and look down in the mouth,
maybe hunched shoulders, will "plonk" him or herself down
heavily on a chair with arms folded, chin on chest and withdraw from
verbal communication. Inside the mind, festering angry thoughts
are mulled over and over and a downward spiral develops as the

thoughts provoke more reminders and more resentment and self-pity. Willow is the remedy to lift people out of this gloomy mood and help them to see life in a brighter light, more optimistically and happily.

VINE people, on the other hand, are not generally likely to sulk. If they are told off or feel humiliated, they are strong enough to stand up for themselves and so will answer back and stand their ground. They hate to be told what to do or feel that someone has got the better of them, and will fight back to regain their dominant position. This can cause them to be aggressive and bullying in their approach, although if their assertiveness and strong will is channelled positively, they can be extremely good leaders. They detest being subservient, yet are obliged to put up with *being* in that situation because school, home and society hold a more commanding role. The Vine remedy helps them to be patient and use their time at school to learn as much as they can, to accumulate all the knowledge gained during their growing years, so that they are able to put it to good use in adult life to fulfil their ambitions and take a leading role in society.

Frustration is so often caused by not being understood; speaking your mind and feeling as though you are speaking to a brick wall because no-one listens to what you have to say. VERVAIN is the remedy for this kind of frustration and the feelings of injustice, being upset by unfair attitudes, such as cruelty, ill-treatment of animals and other issues. Adolescents are beginning to explore life as a whole as well as personal matters, and so form opinions about things that matter to them, and Vervain people feel *very* strongly about these issues. The remedy helps them to relax so that they can approach problems calmly and rationally.

For those who are irritable, quickly lose patience and have a very short temper, IMPATIENS is indicated. It is for those who get frustrated if something does not happen quickly enough and are tempted to snatch or hasten a conversation if it is progressing too slowly for their quick and agile mind. The Impatiens remedy has a calming influence, enabling the mind to work at a more relaxed pace – always astute, but not so rushed, so that there is time for enjoyment and appreciation of the moment. The remedy thus helps to curb the quick temper that suddenly ignites at the slightest irritation.

BEECH is the remedy for the "annoyed" teenager; it is for intolerance which may be directed at parents, brothers, sisters, society or life generally. Things get on the nerves. People's habits aggravate and irritate. The adolescent only sees his or her mother or father's faults and forgets all their good points; criticises them for slurping their tea or for the way they dress. Nothing pleases the Beech. They cannot understand and have no empathy for anything that does not fit in with their own ideas. The Beech remedy helps to bring about a greater appreciation for others, an understanding that we *all* make mistakes, that everyone is different, unique and special in their own way, and that everyone has something individual to offer.

Many teenagers have a lot of love to give, but sometimes that love turns inward and becomes a selfish and possessive self-love, leading to a yearning for attention and craving to be noticed. CHICORY helps those who do not like to let go, who hold on to friends, cling to relationships and drain them of love. Chicory people thrive on love, but the remedy helps them to channel it more constructively – to appreciate that other people cannot be manipulated and controlled like puppets, to respect their independence and learn to let go, welcoming a loving relationship but allowing other people the freedom to live their own lives too.

Some adolescents have a very rigid outlook which causes tension and strict resolve, forcing excessive competitiveness and determination to be the best in the class, or the fastest runner in the school etc. It is this frame of mind that is the driving force behind continued long silences, stubbornly refusing to speak or make up after a row. ROCK WATER helps those of this nature to relax enough to enjoy the pleasures in life as well as the challenges.

IV | **SUICIDE** | Keeping up with life, with peers and with society's expectations can, for some boys and girls, be very hard. They feel under pressure with the responsibility of life generally or unhappy with some element of it. Keeping up appearances with friends forces many to keep smiling and put on a brave face in order to join in with everyone else, but this pretence hides a deepening depression.

Some have such a realistic mask that no-one realises that it is a façade. They truly believe that the personality they see is an accurate reflection of the character underneath. This is sadly why so many of these apparently happy people become desperately depressed and may, as a result, attempt suicide. In many cases it is a cry for help and not a real wish to die, but for others, life seems so empty that they really feel there is nothing at all to live for.

Remedies to help someone experiencing such an unhappy time should be directed at the individual's expression of depression: AGRIMONY if the true feelings are kept well hidden, if they only *appear* to be happy and content; SWEET CHESTNUT for the awful despair and anguish; CHERRY PLUM for uncontrollable suicidal urges; WILLOW for intense self-pity, believing nobody loves them and that the world is so against them that life is no longer worth living; GORSE for those who feel so hopeless that they give up on life altogether.

There are numerous reasons why a teenager might feel this way – broken relationships, bereavement, lack of friendship, being unable to do school-work, feeling a failure and many many more. Some remedy possibilities have been given here, but they are only examples of what might be appropriate. Everyone is different and so one needs to assess the needs on an individual basis.

Whatever reasons a person has for trying to take their own life, it is a tragedy that they should be so unhappy that they feel this is their only way out. Unfortunately we do not always know how a person is feeling because they do not tell us, and a painted smile can be so deceiving that the tears that fall inside are never noticed. If however, we do see through the mask, then the appropriate remedies can help to relieve the state of mind with which these girls and boys are troubled, and help them to see that life is worthwhile after all, before it is too late.

BEST FRIENDS

Most children acquire one particularly close friend. They pal up with another child with whom they get along, and then stick together. Best friends, however, seem to come and go, easily replaced if they should fall out or be parted for some reason. In adolescence, best friends seem to be more important for girls than for boys because girls often have such a close and personal approach to life that it is important and reassuring to have someone to relate to and share it with. Boys have best friends too, but they do not usually demonstrate such close attachment.

Best friends are like soul-mates, substitute sisters or brothers and a special, exclusive rapport develops between them. Girls (or boys) who are popular with their peers may be sought after as good best-mate material, and whoever is chosen may become the object of much jealousy, especially from the redundant last best-friend! HOLLY is the remedy for jealousy should this be a problem. CHICORY would help those who find it hard to let go and so try to hold on to any remaining links that used to tie them together. A mixture of the two remedies would help the girl who feels hurt, jealous and revengeful. WILLOW would be the remedy for the girl who becomes bitter and sulky with self-pity.

Close friendship, however, does provide a certain amount of moral support, but when one of the two friends is left alone if, for example, one is ill or on holiday, the one remaining may be very lonely and feel that she no longer has the same degree of confidence or strength as she did when her companion was there acting as a reassuring prop. It is at a time like this when self-doubt, self-consciousness and vulnerability creep in, when a girl wishes to goodness that she had a wider circle of friends. This is especially so for the girl who is the quieter of the two, as she would draw strength from her extrovert and confident counterpart.

If the separation is to be permanent, the initial wrench may be like a bereavement, leaving the remaining girl feeling utterly lost without her friend. STAR OF BETHLEHEM would help to overcome her grief, and WALNUT would help her to adjust and start again. If she is dwelling too much on the past, HONEYSUCKLE would help, or WILLOW if she feels sorry for herself and mooches around with a "long" face. LARCH will help her to feel more confident; CERATO will help her believe in herself; GENTIAN will help her to be more positive about the future, and MIMULUS will help her to overcome her shyness.

Adolescence is a normal stage of development. We all go through it in our own way, and experience varying degrees of upheaval, yet there remains a common pattern that follows on from one generation to the next. It is a learning period for us all, whether we are parents of teenagers or working with young people, and although it can present certain difficulties, adolescence need not be full of storm and stress or create bad feeling and rejection. It can just as well become a great bonding period, getting to know one another, and accepting each other as fellow adults. Allowing that generation gap, which is very often ultimately responsible for the "problem" in the first place, to close will help parents and their adolescent sons and daughters become friends instead of enemies.

CHAPTER 10

Looking Towards the Future

I | **EXAMINATIONS** | Approaching the end of the compulsory school years, means that final examinations are imminent. Whatever girls or boys want to do afterwards – stay on at school, go to college, go into training for a trade, or just leave to get a job in order to earn some money to enable them to lead an independent life – examinations have to be overcome first, and whatever lies ahead, passing them will help in their quest for a fulfilling career.

For some, passing the examination is not enough, they have to pass it well, because obtaining certain grades is crucial to the requirements of what they want to do. For others, who may not have such a clear idea set in their mind, the exams may represent an inconvenient hurdle and nothing more.

Unfortunately, the age at which these important examinations take place is the same age that adolescents are often least appreciative of their value – everything else is infinitely more interesting! Studying each night when they could be going out enjoying themselves is not an option easily taken. Some will do so fervently because they want to do well and are therefore willing to sacrifice some fun in order to get through their exams successfully. Others may make an entirely different choice and reject study in favour of fun and leisure. In both cases, however, there will be those who make their choice unwillingly or unhappily. Those who want to study may struggle to achieve, and others who *could* do well may not have the confidence to believe in their own success. The remedies can be of great help at examination times, and this will apply whatever level the exams might be because the associated emotions will be the same.

PROCRASTINATION – HORNBEAM is the remedy that is needed when a person keeps putting things off, feeling too tired to drum up the motivation to begin studying, always thinking of something more interesting they could or should be doing. The Hornbeam remedy helps them to overcome this feeling of weariness and be able to tackle their work with greater pleasure.

SELF-CONFIDENCE – LARCH will help those who lack the confidence in themselves to believe that they will pass the examination. If they doubt themselves too much they may not feel it is worth trying and so miss out on the opportunity. Larch people often *have* the ability, but they do not believe it of themselves. The remedy therefore helps them to have more faith.

DISCOURAGEMENT – GENTIAN is for disappointment, discouragement and depression due to a set-back. If a person who is trying to achieve cannot understand a particular topic, or receives a low mark, then Gentian will give the encouragement needed to bounce back and try again.

APATHY – WILD ROSE is for those who lack motivation and enthusiasm for anything beyond what they have already. The Wild Rose type of person is content with life the way it is and does not particularly wish to do anything striking to change it. However, at times, even Wild Rose people can feel they are becoming too apathetic and that life is passing them by – opportunities are lost and they realise, often too late, that they have missed out. The remedy helps such people to take stock of their life and to grasp it in both hands so that they are *not* left behind.

"EXAMINATION NERVES" – RESCUE REMEDY is the most appropriate remedy and extremely helpful when the examination is so close that it begins to create tremendous anxiety – the familiar "butterflies" in the tummy, panic at the last minute and so on. Panic at a time when a clear head and stable thoughts are vital can be disastrous, so Rescue Remedy given at frequent intervals prior to the examination – the days leading up to it, if necessary, as well as the morning itself – can be extremely comforting and beneficial on these stressful occasions.

DISQUIET – ASPEN is also helpful for the apprehension that often accompanies panic, fear and loss of control. It would therefore be a helpful remedy to take in addition to Rescue Remedy. It is for the type of fear and anxiousness that is for no definite reason, and although the cause of the fear in this case is *known,* – the examination itself – there is sometimes an unexplained reason for it too. For example, a person may be confident and know that he or she can do well, and yet have a strange sense of uneasiness and impending disaster. Aspen helps to stem this uncomfortable anxiety.

Studying hard and for long periods can be mentally draining, especially when a series of examinations are being taken and study has to take place in-between sitting individual exams. OLIVE is the remedy for exhaustion and would help to relieve the brain-numb feeling and replenish lost energy. Rest is vital in order to have a clear head for the examination. Sometimes being over-tired can prevent sleep from being refreshing and may even cause insomnia. WHITE CHESTNUT would help to relieve persistent worrying thoughts and mental arguments that are frequently associated with sleeplessness, but sometimes simply relieving the exhaustion (Olive) will help the person to relax enough to drift into sleep and feel refreshed, and wake with restored vitality to face the next stage of the procedure. Olive would also be useful to have on hand afterwards because exams can be so mentally taxing that many students emerge completely drained.

Once the examinations are over, the remedies may not be required again – that is, until the results are due! Once again, the feelings of panic may be apparent, so RESCUE REMEDY would be useful. Hopefully the results will be positive, and result in joy and celebration, but sadly there are bound to be some who receive disappointing news and so the remedies will again prove to be a tremendous comfort. GENTIAN is the most obvious choice for the disappointment, but if there is loss of hope altogether and he or she becomes pessimistic about trying again, then GORSE would be more appropriate. LARCH would help to revive flagging confidence, and WILLOW would help those who sulk and get into a resentful mood, feel very sorry for themselves and express bitterness at their "failure".

Both ROCK WATER and VERVAIN people are perfectionists and they can both force themselves to work extremely hard. Vervain find strength from their enthusiasm and they usually enjoy what they are studying, get involved in it because they have a genuine interest. They can, however, overwork and become tense as a result. Rock Water people strive for perfection within themselves, not because they are necessarily enthusiastic about what it is they are setting out to achieve, but because it represents a test of their strength and stamina. They set themselves a target and go to great lengths to reach it. They too can overwork yet at the same time, rather enjoy the self-sacrifice and challenge. The remedies help people of these respective natures to relax which in turn enables them to be calmer and less demanding in their approach, and this will ultimately help them to achieve their aims and ambitions with less related stress. If they should fail (although it does not happen very often with these people), they will both be understandably upset. Having worked so hard with nothing to show for it will be very difficult to come to terms with. **Vervain** may become incensed with questions and queries as to *why* he or she failed, genuinely interested in order to address the problem and pass next time round (although they may also need LARCH and GENTIAN to help them regain their confidence and overcome their doubt). **Rock Water** people tend to become self-punishing and get annoyed with themselves for having "failed" by only achieving a second degree mark, which may to most people, be considered extremely good. However, second best is not for the Rock Water, and so they set even stricter targets and harsher rules in their attempt to achieve absolute perfection.

Sometimes teenagers can feel under tremendous pressure – due to, as they see it, the expectations of teachers, friends or their parents. They may feel that they have to do as well as their brother or sister and that nothing less than this will do. If they do not achieve that standard they feel a failure and believe that they have let everyone down, including themselves. ROCK WATER would help those who are unrealistic in what they are aiming to do. OLIVE would help the tiredness that an enforced amount of work can create. GENTIAN for the dismay, and ELM for the overwhelming sense of pressure and responsibility that the desire to do well can cause. CERATO would be a useful remedy for those who need constant approval to support them in all they do. The remedy will give them faith and enough trust to overcome their sense of foolishness.

II | **ON THEIR WAY TO WORK...** | Some people have very clear ideas about what they want to do in life. Others really have no idea and can see no further than the end of schooling. Some simply do not care. However they may feel about it, one thing is certain – the future *will* arrive and so the time will come when they need to look for a job, and work for the best part of the rest of their life.

Bearing in mind that we spend more waking hours at work than anywhere else, it makes sense to aim to do something that is both enjoyable and offers job satisfaction. In an ideal world we would all be working vocationally, looking forward to it, doing something with meaning, something that was a pleasure. Unfortunately we do not live in an ideal world, and even if we did, there would always be jobs that were routine, boring and soul destroying.

To some extent it is up to us to decide what we want to do with our lives but there are many angles to approaching work, and we certainly do not always get what we aim for. In the beginning, there is a choice of staying on at school to take advanced exams with perhaps a view to going on to university or college, or of leaving school and looking for work straight away. That decision can be a tough one because a tug of war often goes on between what the heart wants to do and what the head thinks it ought to do. Staying on in full-time education would provide an opportunity to gain higher qualifications with eventual expectations of work that is both financially rewarding and enjoyable. On the other hand, to leave school, forget about study and instead have the freedom to earn enough money to be independent, go out, have fun, dress up and so on, can be very tempting.

Arriving at the right decision may provoke a great deal of mental torment as advantages are weighed up over disadvantages. The remedy to help the way ahead seem clearer and thus make the decision easier is SCLERANTHUS. If however, once the choice has been made, there is doubt over whether it is right, and is followed by a question and answer session with virtually *everyone,* in an attempt to solve the problem, the remedy required would be CERATO.

For those who want to do something of worth or who have ambition but are unable to decide what path to take in order to achieve the fulfilment they seek, WILD OAT is the remedy to help the way forward appear clearer. It helps one find direction in life, and is therefore a very useful remedy whenever a cross-roads like this is reached.

The employment market varies a great deal, and depends a lot on geographical location, political policy, the economy and the demand for a particular trade or the manufacture of certain goods. Some years see a boom in trade and industry, and in response, plenty of job opportunities, but in other years there is a decline, recession and increased *un*employment. Job hunting can, therefore, with the best will in the world be extremely depressing. Searching un-successfully, going to one interview after another and being repeatedly turned down is understandably demoralising. The remedy GENTIAN, although it cannot provide a much wanted job, can help to replace lost faith with hope, and give encouragement to try again. If the despondency is much deeper than this, GORSE may be more appropriate as it is the remedy for those who have lost *all* hope and who have become so pessimistic that they give up trying. WILD OAT can help here too, for those who feel they are going round in circles, applying and being interviewed for jobs that are of little interest to them, and finally begin to wonder why they have applied for them at all, yet at the same time unable to think of anything better.

WILD ROSE would help those who, unlike the Wild Oat, do not feel sufficiently motivated to even consider what they might really like to do, but instead, accept whatever is going, whether it be an interesting job, tedious job or no job at all. Wild Rose would help such people to be more interested in life so that they do not waste their talents.

Although the idea of 24 hours a day of spare time may seem attractive at first, in reality, unemployment is extremely boring because whilst there are all sorts of things one *could* do, given the opportunity, financial restrictions make doing them impossible. A job means money, money means doing the things you want to do, and so without a job, life can be exceedingly monotonous.

Boredom can result in frustration for a number of people, who then try to provide their own entertainment by doing mischief. It may all start unintentionally, an innocent idea or experiment that gets out of hand, and so as a result of boredom, young people may find themselves in trouble with the police, perhaps having made some sort of public nuisance or stolen money or been caught shoplifting... anything to relieve the monotony. If the experience seems exciting then it is likely to be repeated, and a vicious circle may soon develop. Remedies that could be helpful in this situation are dependent on the personality and individual response. HOLLY and VINE would help those who have a revengeful attitude, lash out at society and rebel against its moral values, to channel their energies constructively rather than destructively. It is however, even more important to consider prevention rather than cure and tackle the boredom or frustration from the outset. Some likely suggestions are as follows:

DISINTEREST – CLEMATIS for those who have little interest in what is going on *now;* those who focus their thoughts on the future – what is *going* to happen or what *might* be lying round the corner. Clematis people become bored with the present because of their pre-occupation with what is to come. They can be so bored that they will be constantly tired, sleep a great deal, yawn a lot and be generally drowsy. It may also be used as a form of mental escapism, blotting out the mundane events of everyday life in favour of a future fantasy. The Clematis remedy will not remove their unique imagination, but will help them to be aware of the present too, and feel more grounded in their approach to life *now,* so that they do not miss out on what it has to offer.

TENSION – VERVAIN is for those who are enthusiastic about life, but are frustrated because they are held back. They are people who enjoy a challenge and have ambition but if unable to express it become tense and angry. The Vervain remedy helps to relieve the tension and frustration so that looking for work, and life generally, can be approached more calmly and rationally.

RESENTMENT – WILLOW would help those who blame society for causing unemployment, and for their failings, and believe that everyone and everything is wrong. It is for sulkiness, self-pity and bitterness with life. The remedy helps those who feel this way to look ahead more optimistically, and realise that no one person or action is to blame, and so help them look out of themselves and realise that the world in which they live is not as miserable as it seems.

FEAR – MIMULUS – this would help relieve the fear of long-term unemployment, the fear of poverty, of being disowned, branded as lazy and so on. Any known fear calls for the Mimulus remedy, which helps to replace nervousness with courage.

SELF-DOUBT – LARCH – trying to get a job and constantly failing in each attempt, can make even the most confident person begin to lose self-esteem. Larch therefore is the remedy for anyone who needs to re-gain their self-confidence, especially those who had little to begin with and now find that not only have they no confidence left, but are fast losing their self-respect as well. The remedy is reassuring and as it bolsters confidence, acts as a reminder of the person's true value and talent.

RESILIENCE – OAK is for those who, no matter what adversity is thrown at them, never lose heart, and never give up. They struggle on regardless and are therefore admired as a pillar of strength. There is nothing negative in this and no need as such for the remedy. However, these people are inclined to try *too* hard, and become over-tired and then may begin to lose the strength they once had. The loss of strength causes a great deal of dissatisfaction and frustration, and it is then that the Oak remedy is required. It helps the person recover and re-build their inner determination.

WORRY – WHITE CHESTNUT would help to ease worries about being jobless, or worries about the job itself. It is the sort of worry that causes a person to lie awake at night, the mind over-active and unable to "switch off". The White Chestnut remedy helps to give the sufferer peace of mind and so calms and comforts and helps to contain the thoughts so that the problem can be looked at more objectively and clearly.

REMORSE – PINE would help those who feel guilty about not living up to expectations or for letting other people down. Many teenagers who appreciate their parents' support during their education, and have looked forward to being successful so that their parents will be proud of them, may feel desperately guilty if they are unable to find a job. They may feel useless, worthless and condemn themselves for being a waste. They may feel guilty because they have not achieved good enough examination results, and blame themselves because they should have tried harder. Maybe they *could* have tried harder, but that is beside the point. The Pine remedy helps these people put their feelings into a more realistic perspective so they can appreciate that what has gone has gone, that they must now look forward, and that there is no need to reprimand themselves for something that really cannot be helped. HONEYSUCKLE would also help those who are full of regrets.

LETHARGY – HORNBEAM helps those who feel they lack the strength to face the day ahead, who wake up in the morning, pull the covers back over their head and wish they could cancel the day altogether. If a person has been unlucky in finding employment, they may well feel in this lethargic state, but it can happen when one is in work too – being unable to face going to work, wishing that it was time to come home again, hoping that something will happen to excuse them and enable them to put it off until tomorrow… The Hornbeam feeling usually disappears once the day or task is actually in progress, but it can be very helpful in actually establishing the frame of mind that is conducive to getting up and going to work, or getting up to look for work.

ADAPTATION – WALNUT helps to prepare the young person for leading life as an adult by helping them to adjust to the change of leaving the security and established routine of school to the uncertainty and challenge of the world of work. There is a lot to get used to – people's attitudes, working for others and pleasing them rather than working solely for the development of one's own interest, getting used to taking responsibility, working as a team, handling money and so on. These all represent new challenges which can be disorientating, if not frightening. Walnut helps the young person to adapt more easily. If they should feel overwhelmed with the responsibility of this new life, then ELM would help too.

A LIFE OF THEIR OWN

Parents sometimes worry if their son or daughter seems intent on apparently wasting their life by striving towards something that they do not believe there can be any fruitful future in – pursuing art with the desire to be a famous painter; fashion, wanti..g to be a sought after designer or model; music, intent on becoming a musician, play in an orchestra or form a band; sport, wanting to be a footballer or Olympic athlete... Many parents consider these pursuits to be fanciful and dismiss them as only hobbies, and not a serious consideration for a working future. Whilst in some ways, these ambitions may be based on imaginative hopes and dreams with only the remotest chance of success, one cannot dismiss a person's desire to have something more than a mundane job that, no matter how secure it may be, offers little scope for creativity. If a young person has a yearning to excel at what they are good at and what they enjoy doing, then whether they do actually achieve the pinnacle of their ambitions or not, at least they will be meeting a need within themselves, and that is important when forming a foundation on which a lifetime's happiness, fulfilment and satisfaction is to stand. With encouragement and the right opportunities, those gifts can be channelled in the right direction, so offering every chance to make their dreams come true.

Life is a series of changes and new challenges, and the childhood and adolescent years are packed to the brim with change after change. The remedies will help us all to cope with the problems that life sets in our path, and they are especially important for the teenager who is travelling through the most potentially exciting years of his or her life. It would be a great shame not to enjoy them, and by using the remedies to help your teenagers through the traumas they are bound to meet along the way, they will have every chance of being happy and gaining all they can from their teenage years so that they have a hopeful and happy future to plan and look forward to.

IV	AND FINALLY...

Bringing up a child is hard work, but it can be enormous fun too. Nearly everyone has their own expectations and mental picture of what life will be like when the baby is first born, yet rarely does the reality of it echo what they have imagined. Sleepless nights, disrupted evenings, constant demand for attention and amusement… and then when the child grows up, the moodiness and rebellion associated with adolescence.

Many parents wonder where on earth they have gone wrong and are convinced that they must have faltered somewhere along the way, feel guilty for any problems the child may face and blame themselves for deviancy during the teenage years. However, no matter how much you might condemn yourself for being a "dreadful" mother or father, there is never usually anything to feel guilty about because the negative stages are common to *all* children, albeit in greater and lesser degrees, and whilst of course, there are external pressures and influences that no doubt contribute to unruly behaviour, most young people are just experiencing what is normal and natural.

The remedies are there to help the traumas of growing up be that much easier to cope with, and by doing so, not only make the child or adolescent's life happier and more peaceful, but also have a secondary calming influence on your own life because if you have happy kids, then you stand a good chance of establishing and maintaining a happy home environment.

Parents often forget their own needs because they are too anxious about their children to worry about themselves. However, your own feelings and state of mind are important and should not be neglected. The remedies are there to help you too, and I feel sure that if you have not found so already, there will be moments when you really do feel you could do with a helping hand. There will be occasions when you worry, feel hurt, concerned or frustrated, and as with other things in life, these emotions can begin to snowball if you are not careful. The remedies will not wave a magic wand and solve all your problems, but they will help you to cope and stay on top of it all.

There will be a rapid succession of changes for the child, but there is a great deal for the parents to get used to as well and one of the biggest things to come to terms with is the child growing up. As babies, your children are entirely dependent upon you but suddenly they are no longer infants, they discover their autonomy and want to be independent. The little child that you have nursed and tended to all those years seems, almost overnight, to have gone through some form of metamorphosis and emerged as an independent individual who rejects you as a parent, scorns your advice, questions your motives and treats you as though you have been asleep all your life and know nothing about anything! This is when most parents wonder where they have gone wrong, and can be left feeling bewildered and terribly upset as though a door has slammed in their face.

However negative it might seem at times, however, one small comfort is that you are not alone. There are thousands upon thousands of other parents out there experiencing the same traumas, just as there are thousands upon thousands of other children and teenagers also sharing similar ups and downs. Although this book has dealt mainly with problems and disturbances, this is because the Bach Remedies are intended to help relieve the negative aspects of life, but everything has a positive side too, and by and large, bringing up a family will have far more positive, bright and happy periods than those that cause tears and disharmony.

Bringing a child into the world and watching it grow is a gift of life, something to cherish and be thankful for. It also provides a wonderful opportunity to open a new chapter in your own life, offering you the chance to experience a host of exciting new challenges. It is a period of growth, development and learning for you all, and if you allow yourself to grow *with* your child, you will reap a warm and satisfying relationship.

"*Health is our heritage, our right. It is the complete and full union between soul, mind and body; and this is no difficult far-away ideal to attain, but one so easy and natural that many of us have overlooked it.*

Our souls use our minds and bodies as instruments, and when all three are working in unison the result is perfect health and perfect happiness.

Our mission means no sacrifice, no retiring from the world, no rejecting of the joys of beauty and nature; on the contrary, it means a fuller and greater enjoyment of all things: it means doing the house-keeping, farming, painting, acting, or serving our fellow-men in shops or houses. And this work, whatever it may be, if we love it above all else, is the definite command of our soul, the work we have to do in this world, and in which alone we can be our true selves, interpreting in an ordinary materialistic way the message of that true self.

We can judge, therefore, by our health and by our happiness, how well we are interpreting this message.

Our souls will guide us, if we will only listen, in every circumstance, every difficulty; and the mind and body so directed will pass through life radiating happiness and perfect health, as free from all cares and responsibilities as the small trusting child."

Edward Bach, 1932

Suggested Reading

BACH FLOWER REMEDIES

The Twelve Healers & Other Remedies by Edward Bach
   (Dr. Bach's own descriptions of the 38 remedies)

Heal Thyself by Edward Bach *(the philosophy of Dr. Bach's work)*

The Bach Flower Remedies Step by Step by Judy Howard
   (an all-round practical guide to selecting the remedies)

Questions & Answers by John Ramsell *(practical answers to questions
   concerning the remedies, their principles and practice)*

The Illustrated Handbook of the Bach Flower Remedies
   by Philip Chancellor *(in depth descriptions of the 38 remedies with
   colour Bach Flower illustrations)*

Bach Flower Remedies for Women by Judy Howard *(a journey
   through a woman's life and how the remedies can help the emotional
   difficulties encountered along the way – menstruation, pregnancy,
   childbirth, fertility, screening, the menopause, coping with the stresses
   of modern day life etc.)*

Dictionary of the Bach Flower Remedies by Tom Hyne Jones
   (positive and negative aspects of each remedy)

The Medical Discoveries of Edward Bach by Nora Weeks
   *(biography – Dr. Bach's medical career and how he discovered the
   Flower Remedies)*

The Original Writings of Edward Bach compiled from the
   archives of the Bach Centre by Judy Howard & John Ramsell
   *(a collection of Dr. Bach's letters, case notes, stories and other work,
   many reproduced in original script)*

Introduction to the Benefits of the Bach Flower Remedies
   by Jane Evans

The Bach Remedies Repertory by F.J. Wheeler

The Bach Flower Remedies Illustrations & Preparations by Nora Weeks & Victor Bullen

All the above published by The C. W. Daniel Co. Ltd., Saffron Walden, Essex.

The Story of Mount Vernon by Judy Howard *(an account of how Dr. Bach's work has continued – a tribute to his successors Nora Weeks and Victor Bullen. Illustrated in colour)* Printed by The Bach Centre

Bach Flower Therapy by Mechthild Scheffer *(describing the remedies and their spiritual applications)* Thorsons Publishers Ltd. 1990

Rescue Remedy by Gregory Vlamis *(a collection of case histories and testimonies from professional and lay people on the benefits of the Rescue Remedy)* Thorsons Publishers Ltd. 1986/1990

❀ OTHER SUBJECTS

Babywatching by Desmond Morris
Johnathan Cape 1991

Green Babies by Dr. Penny Stanway
Random Century Group 1990

Baby & Child by Penelope Leach
Penguin Books 1979

From Birth to Five Years – children's developmental progress by Mary D. Sheridan
NFER-Nelson Publishing Co. Ltd. 1973

Spontaneous Play in early Childhood by Mary D. Sheridan
NFER Publishing Co. Ltd. 1977

Adolescence by John Conger
Harper & Row Ltd. 1979

How Children Fail by John Holt
Penguin Books 1969

Natural Medicine for Children by Julian Scott
    Gaia Books/Unwin Paperbacks 1990

The Family Guide to Homoeopathy by Dr. Andrew Lockie
    Elm Tree Books/Guild Publishing 1989

Homoeopathic Remedies for Children by Phyllis Speight
    The C.W. Daniel Co. Ltd. 1983

Aromatherapy for Women & Children by Jane Dye
    The C.W. Daniel Co. Ltd. 1992

Rose Elliot's Vegetarian Mother & Baby Book
    Fontana Paperbacks 1984

Useful Addresses

The Dr. Edward Bach Centre
Mount Vernon,
Sotwell, Wallingford,
Oxon. OX10 0PZ
(advice and information about Bach Flower Remedies)

The Dr. Edward Bach Foundation
Dr. Bach Centre,
Mount Vernon,
Sotwell, Wallingford,
Oxon. OX10 0PZ
(education, training and registration of Counsellors in the Bach Flower Remedies)

Bach Flower Remedies Ltd.,
6 Suffolk Way,
Abingdon,
Oxon. OX14 5JX
(local stockists, worldwide distribution and all overseas enquiries)

Nelsons Homoeopathic Pharmacy
73 Duke Street,
London. WIM 6BY
(Nelson homoeopathic and Bach Flower Remedy UK mail order)

A. Nelson & Co. Ltd.,
5 Endeavour Way,
Wimbledon,
London. SW19 9UH
(licensed manufacturers of homoeopathic medicines

British Homoeopathic Association,
27a Devonshire Street,
London. WIN IRJ

National Society for the Prevention of Cruelty to Children
67 Saffron Hill,
London. EClN 8RS

Association of Parents of Vaccine Damaged Children
2 Church Street,
Shipton-on-Stour,
Warwickshire. CV36 4AP

Hyperactive Children's Support Group
71 Whyke Lane,
Chichester,
West Sussex. PO19 2LD

Down's Syndrome Association,
155 Mitcham Road,
London. SW17 9PG

Cystic Fibrosis Trust,
Alexandra House,
5 Blyth Road,
Bromley,
Kent. BR1 3RS

Spastics Society
12 Park Crescent,
London. WIN 4EQ

Royal National Institute for the Blind
224–228 Great Portland Street,
London. WIN 6AA

Royal National Institute for the Deaf
105 Gower Street,
London. WC1

Association of Child Psychotherapists
Burg House,
New End Square,
London. NW3 1LT

Children's Cancer Help Centre
P.O. Box 604
Bristol. BS99 1SW

Index

❧ USING THE INDEX

Each emotion or state listed refers to a Remedy (e.g. aggression to Vine) and under the name of the Remedy you will find entries for various situations in which that emotion may occur. There are many ways of describing feelings such as aggression: anger, animosity, bullying, determination, disruptive behaviour, strong will can all be interpretations of aggression in certain circumstances. To keep the index as clear and concise as possible I have used only the definitions in the list of Remedies on pages 2–13, the main headings listed by the author and a few additions where there is a substantial piece of information.

When using the index please do look up the page reference as the full description of the state that is given there will help you decide exactly which Remedy will suit you.

obesity, 145
obsession, 5, 43, 44 *and see* Crab Apple,
  Heather
Olive, 11–12
  and babies, 23, 24
  and body image, 145
  and breastfeeding, 31, 36
  and comfort, 27
  and examinations, 182
  and hay fever, 103
  and hyperactivity, 79
  and illness, 100, 101, 110
  and menstruation, 135
  and parental disharmony, 87
  and tics, 77
over-activity, 7 *and see* Vervain *see also*
  hyperactivity
over-excitement, 7 *and see* Vervain *see
  also* excitability
over-protection, 92–3 *and see* protective
  instinct
over-tiredness, 27 *and see* Impatiens,
  Olive *see also* tiredness
overbearing nature, 59, 175 *and see* Vine
overwhelming responsibility, 4–5, 168
  and see Elm
overwork, 6, 11–12 *and see* Oak, Olive

P

panic, 5, 12, 13 *and see* Rescue Remedy,
  Rock Rose
parental disharmony, 84–8
past, dwelling on, 10–11 *and see*
  Honeysuckle
perfectionists, 7, 176 *and see* Rock Water
period pains, 134–5 *and see*
  menstruation
pessimism, 10, 157, 168 *and see* Gorse
Pine, 6
  and achievement, 62
  and adoption, 91
  and babies, 23
  and body image, 144
  and breastfeeding, 31, 34
  and child abuse, 95
  and death, 112
  and disability, 147
  and dyslexia, 65
  and illness, 108
  and love, 158

and parental disharmony, 86, 87–8
and pregnancy, 163
and rejection, 89
and sexual experience, 160
and sexual impulses, 151, 153
and special needs, 115, 116, 117
and termination of pregnancy, 162
and work, 188
placidity, 3 *and see* Centaury
play, 49–55
PMT (pre-menstrual tension), 135
possessiveness, 4, 176 *and see* Chicory
potty training, 40–1
pregnancy, 81–3
  in adolescence, 158–3, 160–3
  and see birth
pressure, 4–5 *and see* Elm
pride, 44 *and see* Oak, Water Violet
procrastination, 11, 181 *and see*
  Hornbeam
protective instinct, 7 *and see* Vervain *see
  also* over-protection
puberty, 129–39

R

rebellion, 3, 174–6 *and see* Beech
Red Chestnut, 6–7
  and babies, 24
  and breastfeeding, 31
  and death, 111
  and hyperactivity, 79
  and nightmares, 30
  and rejection, 90
  and siblings, 83
  and special needs, 117
reflection, 10–11 *and see* Honeysuckle
  see also thoughtfulness
rejection, 88–90
remedies
  administration of, 16–18
  selection of, 14–16
remorse, 188 *and see* Pine
repetition, 9–10 *and see* Chestnut Bud
Rescue Remedy, 13–14, 18–19
  and asthma, 106
  and bed wetting, 47
  and birth trauma, 20
  and blindness, 125
  and bullying, 67
  and cerebral palsy, 122

and child abuse, 95
and colic, 35
and death, 111
and eczema, 104, 105
and examinations, 181, 182
and hay fever, 103
and illness, 99–100, 101, 102
and menstruation, 133, 134
and nightmares, 30
and spots, 141
and teething, 38
resentment, 13, 187 *and see* Willow
resilience, 187 *and see* Oak
restlessness, 5, 12–13, 157 *and see*
    Impatiens, White Chestnut
revenge, 10 *and see* Holly
Rock Rose, 12
and asthma, 107
and bed wetting, 47
and bullying, 67
and cerebral palsy, 122
and child abuse, 95
and comfort, 28
and deafness, 128
and death, 111
and illness, 108
and menstruation, 133
and nightmares, 30
and parental disharmony, 85
and rejection, 90
and sexual impulses, 151, 154
and termination of pregnancy, 162
Rock Water, 7
and achievement, 62
and babies, 23–4
and body image, 144
and breastfeeding, 34
and cerebral palsy, 121
and comfort, 28
and communication, 59
and disability, 147
and disturbances revealed through
    play, 53
and dyslexia, 65
and eczema, 105
and examinations, 183
and menstruation, 134
and parental disharmony, 88
and perfectionists, 176
and rejection, 90

and special needs, 117
and stammering, 74
and temper, 57
rocking, 27 *and see* Cherry Plum, White
    Chestnut

S

sadness, 12 *and see* Star of Bethlehem
sarcasm, 3 *and see* Beech
schooldays, 59–60
Scleranthus, 7
and achievement, 62, 63
and bullying, 68
and child abuse, 96
and confusion, 168
and disturbances revealed through
    play, 53
and love, 155
and parental disharmony, 86, 88
and puberty, 129
and sexual impulses, 153
and special needs, 117
and stammering, 74
and tics, 76
and work, 184
self assurance, 8 *and see* Water Violet
self-confidence, lack of, 5, 181 *and see*
    Larch *see also* confidence
self-consciousness, 5–6 *and see* Larch
self-containment, 8 *and see* Water Violet
self-control, loss of, 9 *and see* Cherry
    Plum
self-destructive behaviour, 27, 28 *and
    see* Crab Apple
self-discipline, 7 *and see* Rock Water
self-doubt, 3, 145, 187 *and see* Cerato,
    Elm, Larch
self-hatred, 143 *and see* Crab Apple
self-inflicted injury, 27 *and see* Cherry
    Plum
self-pity, 13 *and see* Willow
self-sacrifice, 144 *and see* Rock Water
selfishness, 4, 176 *and see* Chicory
sexual abuse *see* child abuse
sexual experience, 159–60
sexual identity, 149–50
sexual impulses, 150–4
shock, 12, 13, 95, 108 *and see* Rescue
    Remedy, Star of Bethlehem
showing off, 63 *and see* Agrimony,

DATE DUE

8/7/98			
APR 0 4 2001			

GAYLORD · PRINTED IN U.S.A